THE COMPLETE WEIGH DOWN DIET FOR WOMEN

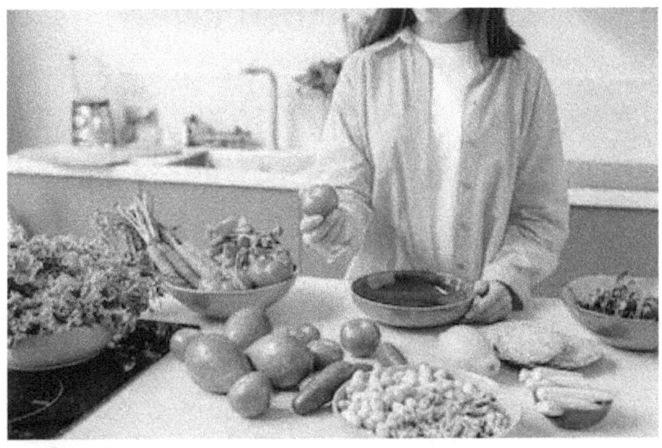

Unveiling a Leaner, Healthier You: The Ultimate Women's Guide to the Weigh-Down Diet

SARAH J. EDWARD

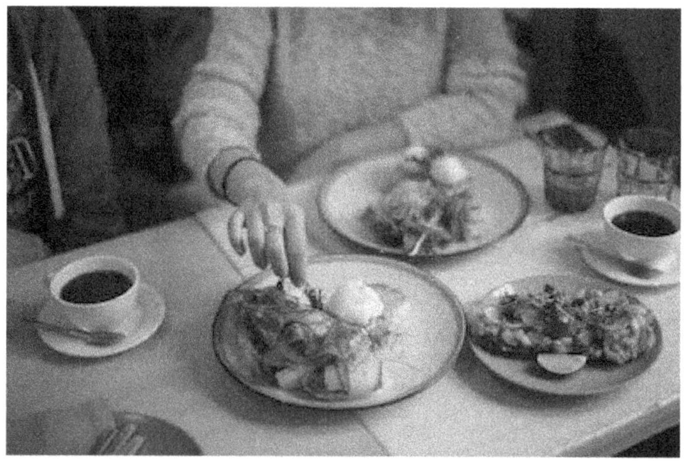

TABLE OF CONTENTS

weight loss include improved mood, increased energy, and overall well-being.

Chapter VI

Overcoming Challenges and Staying Motivated

Common obstacles faced during weight loss journeys and strategies for overcoming them

Tips for managing cravings, dealing with social situations, and staying motivated in the face of setbacks

The importance of self-compassion and the celebration of non-scale victories

Conclusion

Recap the key principles of the Weigh-Down Diet for women

Encouraging readers to embrace a lifelong commitment to their health and well-being

Meal planner

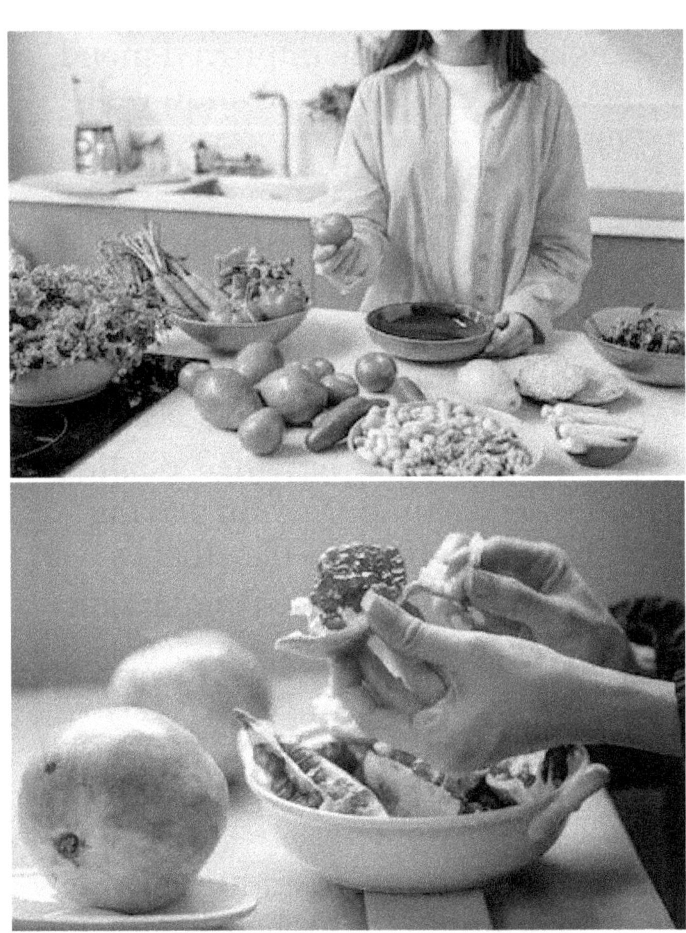

The Complete Weigh Down Diet For Women

DEAR WOMEN,

Please, if you appreciate this book, consider giving it a favorable review, I hope this message finds you well. I'm reaching out to humbly seek your honest evaluation of my book.

*A positive review from one of our honest customers like you makes others feel secure about selecting **"The Complete Weigh Down Diet For Women"**, Sharing your joyful experience will be much welcomed and push me to write more books for your happiness.*

Your review will assist prospective readers and influence their expectations. Your thoughts will be the reason someone chooses to plunge into this literary experience. I'd greatly appreciate your sincere input.

***Thanks** for considering this request.*
Best regards.

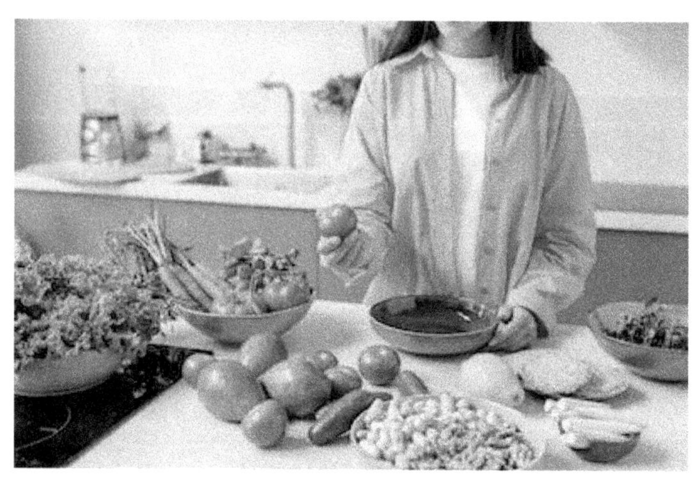

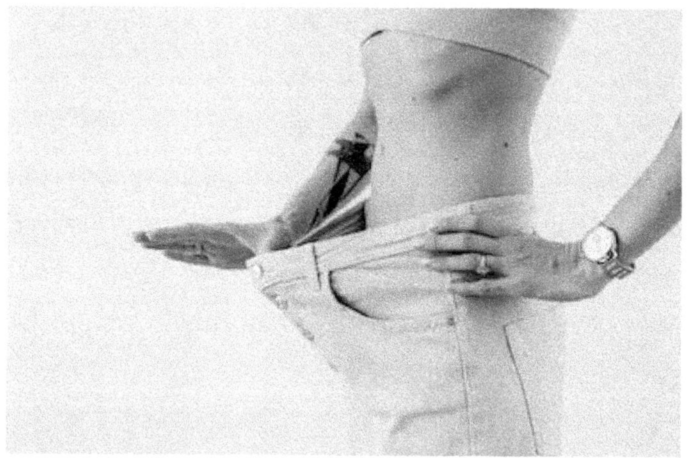

The Complete Weigh Down Diet For Women

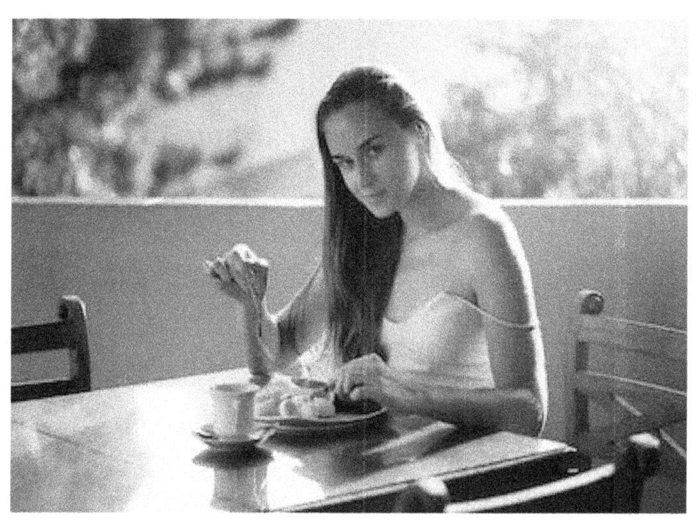

INTRODUCTION

Greetings on your path to a lighter, better, and more confident version of yourself. I urge you to explore the depths of your existence and discover the tremendous power that lives inside you on a fantastic journey through these pages. Together, as we explore the fascinating world of the Weigh-along Diet, we will go along a road of self-discovery, negotiating the physical, mental, and spiritual landscape.

It's easy for women to feel confused and disappointed in a society overrun with fad diets and contradicting weight reduction advice. The quest for the perfect physique often spirals into an unending cycle of deprivation, annoyance, and disillusionment. But what if there was an alternative strategy? What if we could free ourselves from the shackles of unhealthy food and unattainable goals? What if there was a healthy, comprehensive way to lose weight that not only nourished our bodies but also our spirits?

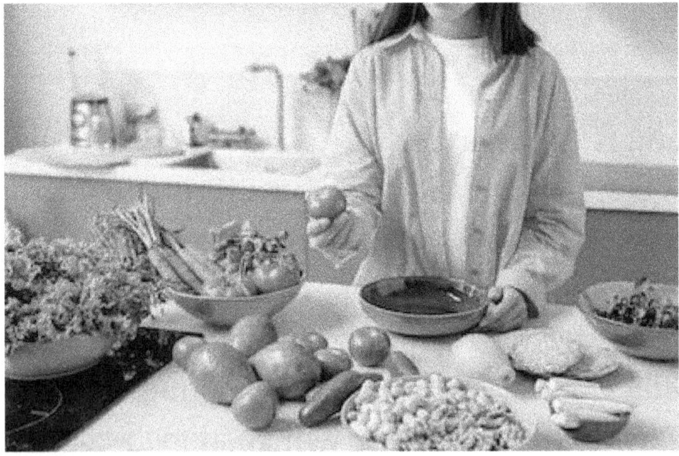

An innovative idea created exclusively for ladies is the Weigh-Down diet. It goes beyond the idea of weight reduction as we know it because it acknowledges the connection between our physical and mental health. It recognizes that our bodies are distinctive storytelling machines, and it gives us the ability to write our own stories.

We shall examine the guiding concepts of the Weigh-Down diet in this book and come to appreciate its capacity for change in our lives. We will examine the fundamental principles of intuitive eating and experience the freedom that comes from paying attention to and respecting our bodies' knowledge.

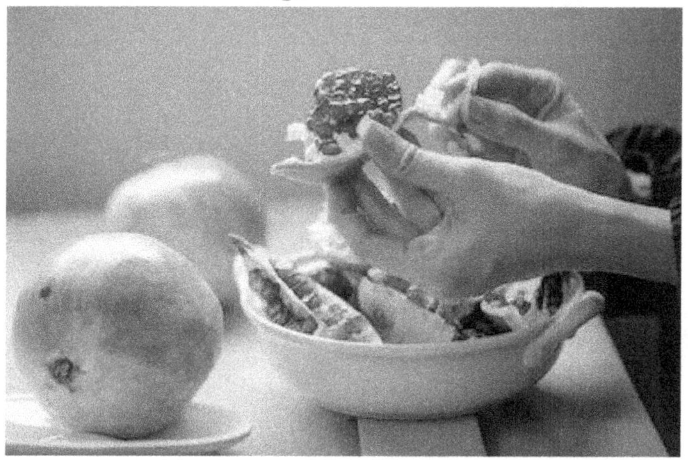

By adopting a clean and balanced approach to eating that nourishes both our bodies and our spirits, we will shed light on the idea of nutrition.

However, this trip is about more than simply the food we consume; it's also about the feelings and self-delusions we carry. We shall set out on a journey of introspection to identify the emotional triggers that have often misled us. We will discover how to embrace self-compassion and forgiveness, enabling us to move beyond our past hurts and into a future that is full of self-acceptance and love.

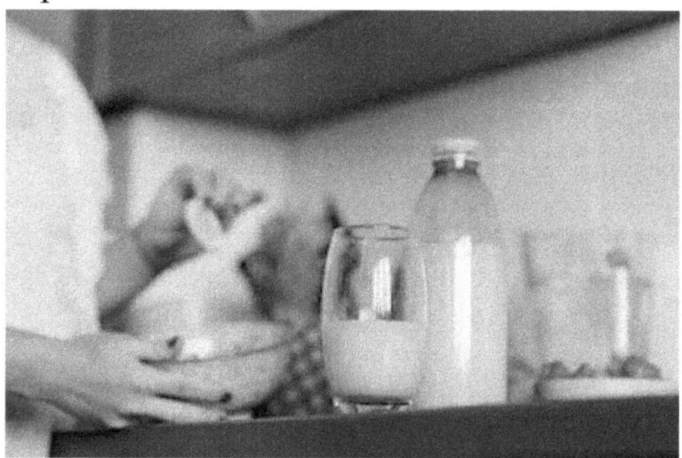

You may discover helpful advice on how to fuel your body with scrumptious, nutrient-dense meals on these pages. We will investigate the delights of menu planning, grocery shopping, and cooking healthful foods that awaken our senses and revitalize our spirits. We will also learn about the importance of movement and find fun ways to include exercise in our everyday routines, not as a chore but rather as a chance to celebrate our bodies and what they are capable of.

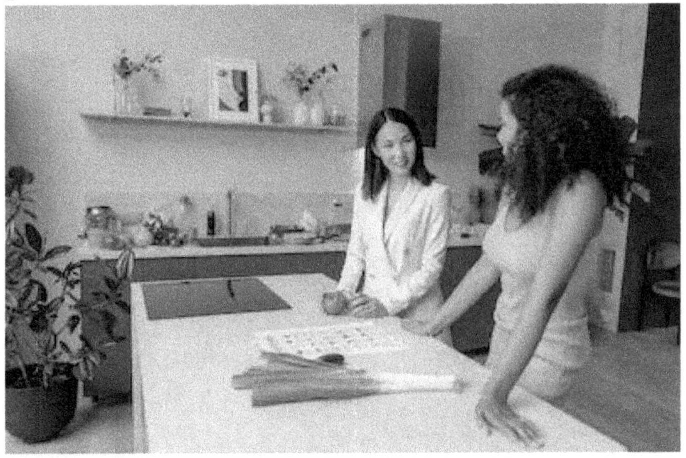

This book is not merely a reference. It is a passionate ally that provides assistance and inspiration at every turn. You will discover inspiration and encouragement to adopt a lifestyle that goes beyond weight reduction and ushers in a new era of thriving health via personal experiences, scientific revelations, and the experiences of women who have already traveled this route.

Kindly note, It is an honor for me to go with you on this remarkable voyage. Let's embrace a life of harmony, joy, and radiant well-being as we reclaim our bodies and rewrite our stories together. I am eager to follow The Lighter Path and see where it leads.

With affection and eagerness,

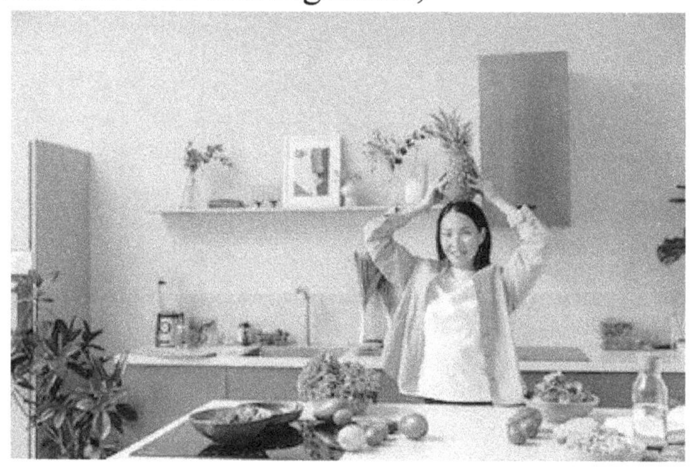

Let get started

The Weigh-Down Diet is a potent and revolutionary technique designed exclusively for women in the crowded field of weight reduction approaches. It serves as evidence for the idea that long-term weight reduction is not just a game of numbers but rather a meaningful journey of empowerment and self-discovery.

The weight-down diet surpasses the limitations of restricted food and fast solutions since it is based on a comprehensive concept. It accepts the interconnectedness of the body and mind, understanding that real change results from nourishing both. This powerful approach centers on intuitive eating, teaching women to respect their own dietary requirements and pay attention to their bodies' intrinsic knowledge.

The Weigh-Down diet promotes a healthy relationship with food that is based on balance and self-compassion, in contrast to conventional diets that encourage deprivation and anxiety. It exhorts women to let go of their guilt and adopt a feeding strategy that nourishes both the body and the spirit.

This novel way of thinking takes into account how strongly emotions affect the way we eat. Women may break the pattern of emotional eating by exploring the emotional triggers that hinder their development, finding consolation in self-reflection, and developing the strength and grace to deal with life's adversities.

There are a wealth of useful tips and techniques included in the Weigh-Down Diet, covering everything from meal planning and grocery shopping to mindful eating and happy activities. It is a thorough manual that equips women with the tools they need to reclaim their bodies, change their attitudes, and begin out on a lifetime path to vibrant health and well-being.

For women looking for a long-term, powerful, and revolutionary method of weight reduction, the Weigh-Down Diet appeals. It is a remarkable path that values uniqueness, encourages balance, and recognizes the limitless potential of every woman. Enter this amazing adventure and release the potential for growth and success that is within you.

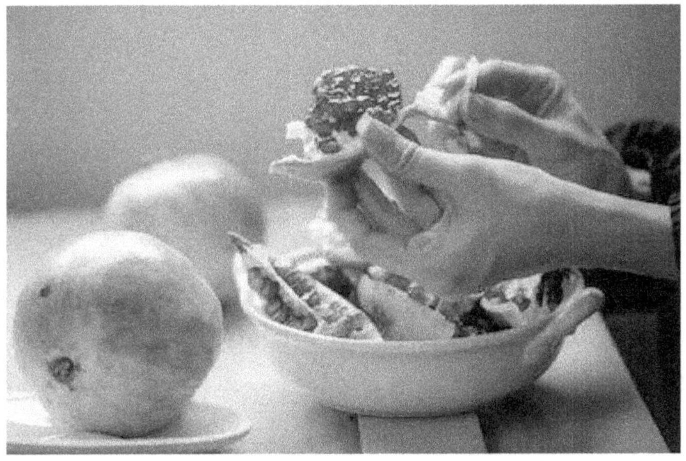

Challenges faced by women when it comes to weight management and body image

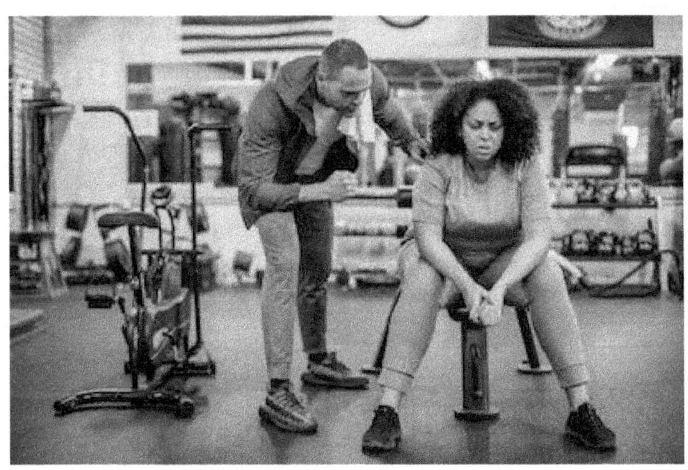

When it comes to body image and weight control, women encounter a variety of difficulties. Figure dissatisfaction and poor self-esteem may be brought on by society's unattainable beauty standards, media portrayals of the "ideal" figure, and social pressures. Additionally, women's attempts to regulate their weight face particular difficulties due to menopause, pregnancy, and hormonal changes. The road is made more difficult by emotional eating, self-comparison, and society's censure. It takes mental change, self-acceptance, and a comprehensive strategy that feeds the body and mind to overcome these obstacles.

Importance of a balanced and realistic mindset towards achieving a healthy weight.

It is impossible to stress the importance of having a sensible and balanced mentality while trying to lose weight. We are much too often subjected to cultural pressures and irrational expectations, which prepare us for letdowns and self-doubt.

A balanced mentality that is balanced understands that taking care of our bodies, brains, and spirits is more important than defining health merely by a weight on a scale. It recognizes that real well-being includes both physical fitness and emotional, mental, and spiritual wholeness.

We liberate ourselves from the hold of fast fixes and unsustainable diets by adopting a realistic perspective. We are aware that real transformation involves effort, perseverance, and consistency. It enables us to establish reasonable objectives, acknowledge tiny accomplishments, and draw lessons from failures.

We may see our bodies with respect and acceptance while recognizing their distinct strengths and flaws when we have a realistic, balanced perspective. It promotes self-compassion, a healthy relationship with eating, and the development of a good self-concept.

Ultimately, we create the groundwork for a lifetime path of wellbeing by creating a balanced and realistic mentality. It helps us adopt a long-term strategy for weight control, resulting in a healthier body as well as a better and more contented life.

Chapter I

Understanding the Weigh-Down Diet

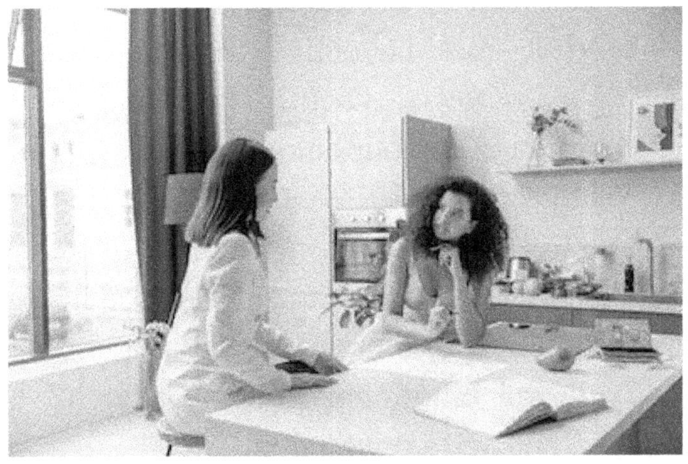

Imagine starting a transformational journey where self-discovery and empowerment guide the way to a better, lighter version of yourself. Greetings from the realm of the Weigh-Down Diet, a wonderful strategy that can help you access your body's intrinsic knowledge and direct you toward long-term weight reduction.

The Weigh-Down Diet's fundamental tenet is intuitive eating, a potent philosophy that exhorts you to pay attention to your body's cues and respect its requirements. No more strict calorie tracking or food planning. Instead, you'll discover how to rely on your gut, enjoy each meal, and take pleasure in feeding your body healthy nutrients.

However, it goes beyond what you consume. The Weigh-Down Diet acknowledges the connection between our emotional state and how we relate to food. We will examine the emotional causes that often result in overeating or unhealthy behaviors together. You'll learn new techniques to nourish your soul and escape the cycle of emotional eating through self-reflection and self-compassion.

Forget about the shame and limitations imposed by conventional diets. You are encouraged to develop a reasonable, balanced mentality through the Weigh-Down diet. You'll set realistic objectives, acknowledge your accomplishments, and learn from failure. It's a path that values your uniqueness and celebrates your dedication to your long-term wellbeing.

Are you prepared to begin this remarkable journey? Be open to the opportunities that lie ahead by widening your heart and intellect. Become the creator of your own health narrative with the help of the Weigh-Down Diet, where freedom, self-discovery, and a lighter you await.

Principles of the Weigh-Down Diet

<u>Imagine this</u>: You're seeking a route that will take you to long-term health and happiness as you stand at the fork in your weight reduction journey. Enter the weight-Down Diet, a revolutionary strategy that goes beyond conventional ideas of weight reduction.

The Weigh-Down Diet, at its foundation, emphasizes a holistic concept, understanding that genuine well-being transcends just the numbers on a scale. It recognizes the connection between our bodies and thoughts and the need to take care of both in order to achieve optimum health.

Physically, the Weigh-Down diet encourages a healthy food philosophy.

It promotes intuitive eating, a strategy that respects our bodies' signals of hunger and fullness. No more imposing strict restrictions or denying ourselves our favorite meals. Instead, we learn to pay attention to our body by mindfully eating, enjoying each mouthful, and feeling satisfied.

The Weigh-Down diet doesn't end with the meal, however. It looks into the emotional side of things and acknowledges how closely related our connection with food is to our emotions. By providing strategies to confront and get over these difficulties, it encourages us to investigate the underlying reasons for emotional eating. By taking care of our mental health, we lay the groundwork for long-term weight reduction and happiness.

So, my friend, the Weigh-Down Diet calls to you if you're ready to choose a diet that feeds both your body and your spirit. Together, we'll set out on a voyage of self-discovery in which food ceases to be only a source of energy and starts to become a source of delight. Prepare to discover the power of a comprehensive strategy, which will open the door to a world of health and pleasure that goes well beyond the scale.

Concept of intuitive eating and its significance in achieving sustainable weight loss.

Imagine living in a society where you could respect the intrinsic knowledge of your body and enjoy your food with freedom. Introducing intuitive eating, a revolutionary idea that may help you lose weight permanently while fostering a positive connection with food.

Fundamentally, intuitive eating encourages you to tune into your body's signals, pay attention to its cues, and treat it with compassion and respect. The era of stringent regulations and outside limitations is over. Instead, you go on a self-discovery journey where you learn to respect the distinct hunger and fullness signals that are exclusive to you.

Eating intuitively goes beyond calorie tracking and portion control. It invites you to enjoy the tastes, textures, and scents of your meals and to take pleasure in the act of mindful eating. It encourages you to develop a stronger connection with your body by acknowledging that it is able to tell you what it needs and when it needs it.

Importantly, intuitive eating acknowledges that success is not just determined by weight reduction. It embraces the idea that health includes physical, emotional, and mental elements and moves the emphasis from numbers on a scale to entire well-being.

You regain control of your life and take control of your body by adopting an intuitive eating philosophy. You discover durable, long-lasting transformation and release yourself from the dieting cycle. It's a ground-breaking strategy that feeds both your body and your spirit, resulting in a healthier, happier, and more peaceful relationship with food and with yourself.

Role of portion control, mindful eating, and finding balance in one's diet

Three important factors—portion management, mindful eating, and achieving balance—come into play while pursuing a balanced and healthy diet. These pillars provide people with the capacity to make thoughtful decisions and have a positive relationship with food.

Portion management acts as a compass, pointing us in the direction of the right amounts. We can prevent overeating and make sure our bodies get the nutrients they need without going overboard by recognizing optimal portion proportions. It enables us to enjoy the tastes and textures of our meals while still paying attention to our bodies' fullness cues.

Engaging all of our senses when eating, mindful eating promotes awareness of the current moment. It nudges us to take our time, enjoy the food before us, and really relish each mouthful. This method deepens our relationship with the food we consume and fosters a greater understanding of how it affects our wellbeing.

Maintaining a healthy and satisfying diet requires finding balance. It entails preparing meals that include a range of food categories, colors, and tastes. By striking a balance between indulgence and moderation, we may sate our appetites while emphasizing nutrient-dense food options. It promotes continued adherence to a healthy lifestyle over time by allowing for flexibility and pleasure, eliminating feelings of deprivation.

We go on a path of self-awareness and empowerment by embracing portion management, engaging in mindful eating, and achieving balance. These ideas help us fuel our bodies, create a lasting feeling of well-being, and establish a positive connection with food.

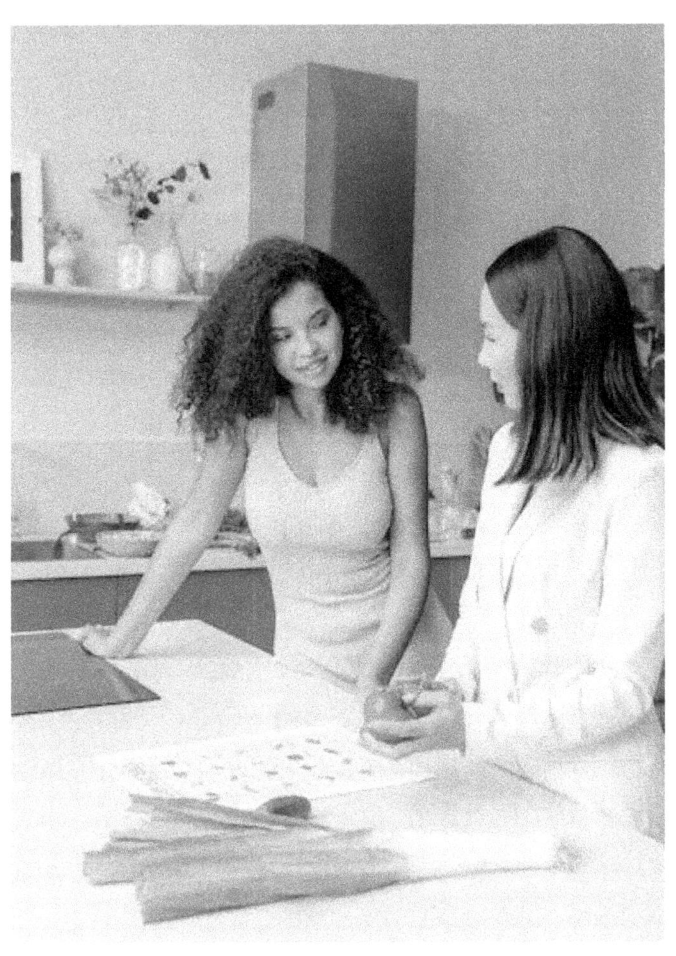

Chapter II

Assessing Your Current Lifestyle

Consider your recent eating habits for a moment. An effective tool for making wise judgments is evaluation. By examining your relationship with food, you may identify areas for improvement and begin a journey of transformation.

Consider your regular meals and snacks critically. Do you eat a variety of nutrient-dense meals? Are you paying attention to your body's hunger and fullness cues? Be sincere with yourself as you consider any established routines of thoughtless nibbling or emotional eating.

By taking an honest look at your eating habits, you could discover a lot about the things that motivate you to make bad food choices. Stress, boredom, or social pressure could play a part. Understanding these patterns enables you to make informed decisions and develop novel solutions to satisfy these essential requirements.

Remember that this evaluation is an opportunity for progress rather than a verdict. Recognize the positive aspects of your current routines while noting the parts that need improvement. Accept your capacity for good judgment and go on a journey to a better and more peaceful relationship with eating.

Practical tips for setting realistic goals and tracking progress

A successful experience on the Weigh-Down Diet depends on setting reasonable objectives and monitoring progress. Here are some helpful hints to help you on your journey:

<u>Clarity comes first:</u> Clearly and fully describe your objectives. Be clear about the goals you have, whether it's losing a particular amount of weight or forming better eating habits.

<u>**Take it apart:**</u> Break down your main objective into more achievable stages. This not only makes your path more attainable but also enables you to recognize little victories along the way.

<u>**Be sensible:**</u> Make sure your objectives are both difficult and doable. Take into account your unique circumstances, obligations, and way of life. Avoid the temptation to aim for quick weight reduction; instead, concentrate on long-term improvement.

<u>**Follow your development:**</u> To keep track of your meals, exercise habits, and eating-related emotions, keep a notebook or use a mobile app. Review and reflect on your entries often to uncover trends, triggers, and areas for development.

<u>**Celebrate accomplishments other than weight loss:**</u> Don't depend exclusively on the scale's reading. Celebrate accomplishments that don't relate to weight, such as more energy, better

sleep, or more comfortable clothing. These triumphs serve as a reminder of the other, more constructive developments taking place.

Adapt and adjust: Be flexible and willing to change your objectives as necessary. Your path is unique to you, and circumstances may change. Accept that you are always growing and changing.

You'll remain inspired and empowered throughout your Weigh-Down Diet journey by establishing realistic objectives and monitoring your progress, assuring long-term success and a rekindled feeling of wellbeing.

The importance of self-reflection and identifying emotional triggers for overeating or unhealthy behaviors

Understanding and dealing with overeating or other harmful habits heavily relies on self-reflection and the ability to recognize emotional triggers. We may learn a lot about the motivations behind our behavior by carefully examining our thoughts, feelings, and habits.

By allowing for introspection and self-awareness, self-reflection enables us to identify the underlying emotions, pressures, or anxieties that motivate us to engage in harmful behaviors. It encourages us to reflect on our ideas and motives, revealing the underlying factors that underlie our conduct.

Finding emotional triggers is important because it reveals the complex link between our emotions and eating patterns. It aids in identifying if we use food as a comfort when we're stressed, bored, lonely, or even as a reward. Knowing these triggers enables us to create healthy coping strategies, increase our emotional resiliency, and foster self-compassion.

We may escape the pattern of thoughtless or emotional eating by reflecting on our behavior and recognizing our emotional triggers. We may create new methods for controlling our emotions and nurturing ourselves in more rewarding ways by addressing the underlying issues. A better connection with food, more self-awareness, and a stronger feeling of control over our well-being are all made possible by this transforming process.

Chapter III

Nourishing Your Body

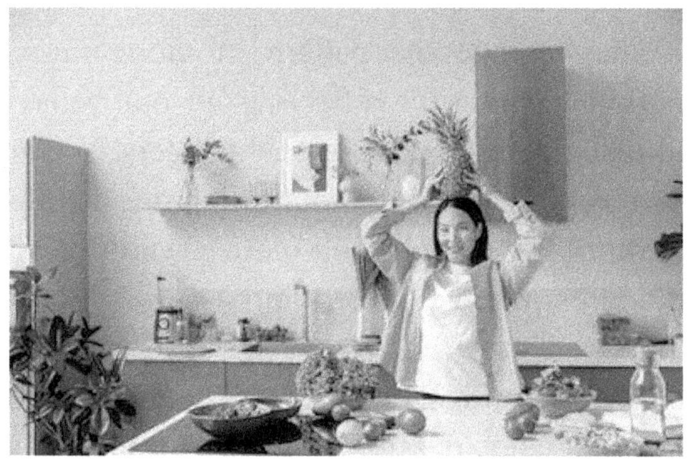

A balanced diet rich in full, nutrient-dense foods is essential to maintaining optimum health and vigor. Such a diet provides our bodies with the vital vitamins, minerals, and antioxidants they need to flourish.

Meal planning, attentive food shopping, and mindful meal preparation are essential if you want to start this wholesome path. We can make sure that our meals are well-rounded and include a range of nutrient-rich products by taking the time to plan them. When we go grocery shopping, we may stock our carts with healthy foods by putting fresh fruits, colorful veggies, lean meats, and whole grains first.

It is possible to increase the amount of these essential ingredients in our everyday meals by taking a few simple but effective actions. We may start by increasing the amount of veggies in each meal, choosing colorful kinds to increase the variety of nutrients. Our intake of fiber is increased and our blood sugar levels are stabilized when we replace refined grains with whole grains like quinoa or brown rice. Lean proteins, such as those found in fish, chicken, and lentils, provide crucial amino acids for muscle repair and general health.

We build a foundation of nutrition that supports our physical and mental health by giving priority to a balanced diet full of whole, nutrient-dense foods. When we take care of our bodies, they flourish with more energy, better digestion, and stronger immune systems. By accepting these options, we set off on a transforming journey in the direction of a lifetime of vigor and wellbeing.

The significance of a balanced diet for women's health and weight control cannot be overstated. The key to sustaining our bodies and encouraging optimum well-being is a diet full of entire, nutrient-dense foods.

Making whole meals a priority allows us to provide our bodies with a wide range of vital vitamins, minerals, and antioxidants that promote good health. Lean proteins feed our muscles and help us feel full, while fruits and vegetables provide a wide variety of minerals and fiber. Whole grains provide you with long-lasting energy and fiber, which is good for your digestive system.

Well-thought-out meal planning, grocery shopping, and meal preparation are essential to incorporating a balanced diet into our daily lives.

Meal planning enables us to choose a range of nutrient-dense items and prepare balanced meals on purpose. When doing your grocery shopping, pay attention to the perimeter of the store, where you'll often find fresh vegetables, lean meats, and healthy grains.

Simple but inventive tactics may be used to include more fruits, veggies, lean meats, and complete grains in everyday meals. Try out vibrant salads, vegetable-packed stir-fries, and filling grain bowls. Make fruit and vegetable smoothies, and enjoy tasty, high-protein dishes like grilled chicken or tofu with nutrient-dense sides.

A balanced diet rich in full, nutrient-dense foods nourishes our bodies, increases energy, and improves our general well-being. Let's go on a gastronomic journey to learn about the delights and advantages of nourishing ourselves with nature's abundance.

Enjoy our weight down recipes

Recipe 1:

Quinoa Salad with Grilled Chicken

Ingredients:

- 1 cup cooked quinoa
- 4 ounces grilled chicken breast, sliced
- 1 cup mixed salad greens
- 1/4 cup cherry tomatoes, halved
- 1/4 cup cucumber, diced
- 2 tablespoons feta cheese, crumbled
- 2 tablespoons balsamic vinaigrette dressing

Instructions:

1. In a large bowl, combine cooked quinoa, grilled chicken breast, mixed salad greens, cherry tomatoes, cucumber, and feta cheese.
2. Drizzle the balsamic vinaigrette dressing over the salad.
3. Toss gently to ensure all ingredients are well coated.

4. Serve immediately and enjoy!

Nutrition per serving:
- ☐ **Calories:** 380
- ☐ **Protein:** 26g
- ☐ **Carbohydrates:** 32g
- ☐ **Fat:** 16g
- ☐ **Fiber:** 4g

Recipe 2:

Veggie Stir-Fry with Tofu

Ingredients:

- 1 tablespoon olive oil
- 8 ounces firm tofu, drained and cubed
- 1 cup broccoli florets
- 1 bell pepper, sliced;
- 1 carrot, julienned
- 1/2 cup snap peas
- 2 cloves garlic, minced
- 2 tablespoons low-sodium soy sauce
- 1 tablespoon sesame oil
- 1 tablespoon sesame seeds (optional)

Instructions:

1. Heat olive oil in a large skillet over medium-high heat.
2. Add tofu cubes to the skillet and cook until golden brown on all sides. Remove from the skillet and set aside.
3. In the same skillet, add broccoli, bell pepper, carrot, snap peas, and minced garlic. Stir-fry for 5-7 minutes or until vegetables are crisp-tender.
4. Return the tofu to the skillet and add soy sauce and sesame oil. Stir-fry for an additional 2-3 minutes, ensuring everything is well coated.
5. Sprinkle with sesame seeds (optional) and serve hot.

Nutrition per serving:

- **Calories:** 280
- **Protein:** 18g
- **Carbohydrates:** 16g
- **Fat:** 18g
- **Fiber:** 6g

Recipe 3:

Baked Salmon with Roasted Vegetables

Ingredients:

- 4 ounces salmon fillet
- 1 cup mixed vegetables (such as zucchini, bell peppers, and asparagus), cut into bite-sized pieces
- 1 tablespoon olive oil
- 1/2 teaspoon dried dill
- Salt and pepper to taste
- Lemon wedges for serving

Instructions:

1. Preheat the oven to 400°F (200°C).
2. Place the salmon fillet on a baking sheet lined with parchment paper.
3. In a bowl, toss the mixed vegetables with olive oil, dried dill, salt, and pepper.
4. Arrange the seasoned vegetables around the salmon on the baking sheet.
5. Bake for 12-15 minutes, or until the salmon is cooked through and the vegetables are tender.
6. Serve with lemon wedges for a fresh citrus flavor.

Nutrition per serving:
- **Calories:** 320
- **Protein:** 24g
- **Carbohydrates:** 12g
- **Fat:** 20g
- **Fiber:** 4g

Recipe 4:

Greek Yogurt Parfait

Ingredients:

- 1 cup plain Greek yogurt
- 1/4 cup granola
- 1/4 cup mixed berries (such as strawberries, blueberries, and raspberries)
- 1 tablespoon honey (optional)

Instructions:

1. In a glass or bowl, layer half of the Greek yogurt.
2. Sprinkle half of the granola on top of the yogurt.
3. Add half of the mixed berries.
4. Repeat the layers with the remaining yogurt, granola, and berries.
5. Drizzle honey on top, if desired.
6. Enjoy this delightful and nutritious parfait as a satisfying breakfast or snack.

Nutrition per serving:

- **Calories:** 220

- ☐ **Protein:** 17g
- ☐ **Carbohydrates:** 26g
- ☐ **Fat:** 6g
- ☐ **Fiber:** 4g

Recipe 5:

<u>Veggie Omelette</u>

Ingredients:

- 2 eggs
- 1/4 cup diced bell peppers
- 1/4 cup diced onions
- 1/4 cup sliced mushrooms
- 1/4 cup baby spinach leaves
- Salt and pepper to taste
- 1 teaspoon olive oil

Instructions:

1. In a bowl, whisk the eggs until well beaten. Season with salt and pepper.
2. Heat olive oil in a non-stick skillet over medium heat.
3. Add bell peppers, onions, and mushrooms to the skillet. Sauté until softened.
4. Add spinach leaves to the skillet and cook until wilted.
5. Pour the beaten eggs over the vegetables, tilting the skillet to spread the mixture evenly.
6. Cook for a few minutes until the bottom is set, then gently flip the omelette.
7. Cook for an additional minute or until the eggs are fully cooked but still tender.
8. Slide the omelette onto a plate and fold it in half.
9. Serve hot and savor the nutritious flavors.

Nutrition per serving:
Calories: 220
Protein: 16g
Carbohydrates: 9g

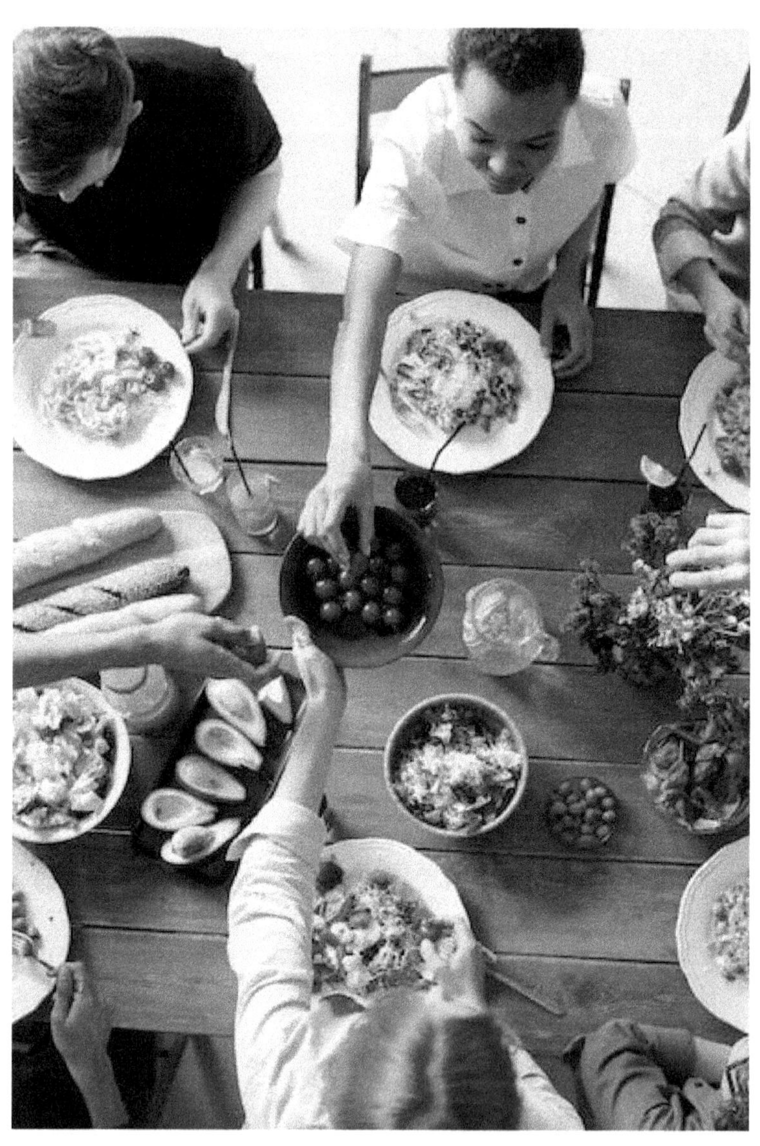

The Complete Weigh Down Diet For Women

Chapter IV

Cultivating a Positive Relationship with Food

The weight-Down Diet places a strong emphasis on developing a healthy connection with food since it paves the way for long-lasting and satisfying eating routines. It entails changing our perspective from seeing food as the adversary to seeing it as a source of gratification, fuel, and sustenance for our body.

We must engage in mindful eating if we want to have a healthy relationship with food. This means enjoying every meal, paying attention to our bodies' hunger and fullness signals, and being completely present and conscious of our eating experiences. We may genuinely enjoy the sustenance our meals bring if we take our time and really pay attention to the flavors, textures, and fragrances they have to offer.

It's essential to give up restrictive diets and adopt a balanced eating philosophy. The goal is to let ourselves indulge in a broad range of meals, especially those we love, without feeling guilty or ashamed. We can make sure our bodies get the vitamins, minerals, and energy they need to flourish by adding a range of nutrient-dense foods to our diet.

Self-compassion is crucial for developing a healthy relationship with food. Instead of blaming ourselves for sometimes indulging in goodies or straying from our eating regimen, we engage in love and empathy. We accept our mistakes and focus our attention on the wider picture of our general health and wellbeing.

Additionally, it's critical to manage emotional eating. It is crucial to identify and accept the emotional triggers that cause us to resort to food for solace. We may interrupt the loop of using food as an emotional crutch by learning new coping skills, such as practicing self-care, asking for assistance from loved ones, or researching stress reduction methods.

In the Weigh-Down Diet, developing a healthy relationship with food entails engaging in mindful eating, accepting balance, growing self-compassion, and addressing emotional triggers. We may create a sustaining and joyful relationship with food that promotes our overall well being by fueling our bodies with purpose, enjoyment, and self-love.

Emotional eating and strategies for overcoming it

An important roadblock on the way to obtaining a healthy weight and a balanced relationship with food might be emotional eating. Food often serves as a comfort or diversion instead of sustenance in reaction to stress, boredom, or other emotional triggers. It is essential to address the underlying emotional demands and create healthy coping mechanisms in order to effectively overcome emotional eating.

Develop mindfulness as a technique for success. We become more aware of our emotions and the factors that contribute to emotional eating by engaging in mindfulness practices. Before grabbing a bite, we should take a moment to consider if our hunger is the result of physiological requirements or psychological urges. Deep breathing exercises and other practices like journaling and meditation may help us become more self-aware and improve our ability to control our emotions.

Another tactic is to create a network of allies. We might feel more accountable and encouraged when we are around kind and encouraging people who support our goals. It might also be helpful to seek the advice of a therapist, nutritionist, or support group that focuses on overcoming emotional eating in order to get insights, skills, and techniques to do so.

Finding alternate coping strategies is also crucial. Redirecting emotional energy and providing better outlets for stress or negative emotions may be accomplished by participating in activities like exercise, hobbies, or relaxation methods. It's critical to recognize the things that make you happy, content, and relaxed and deliberately pick those things instead of emotional eating.

In the end, it takes time and self-compassion to stop emotional eating. It is a path for healing and self-discovery. We may escape the pattern of emotional eating and cultivate a better and more long-lasting connection with food and ourselves by attending to the underlying emotional needs, practicing mindfulness, creating a support system, and discovering alternative coping techniques.

Develop a healthy relationship with food, free from guilt or restriction.

I beg you, my dear readers, to embrace a deep change in your relationship with food in the context of the Weigh-Down Diet. Release the restrictions and shame that have held you back on your path so far. It's time to liberate yourself.

Food is a source of sustenance, pleasure, and joy; it is not your adversary. It has the capacity to both sate your spirit and feed your body. By developing a positive connection with food, you open the door to a universe of harmony and self-acceptance.

Free yourself from the strain of monitoring your diet and keeping track of calories. Instead, enjoy the process of mindful eating while savoring the tastes and sensations that dance on your palate. Pay attention to your body's nudges and respect its signals of hunger and fullness.

Get rid of the idea that certain meals are "good" or "bad" for you. Accept the idea of moderation and let go of the shame that comes with excess. Recognize that nutrition includes not just providing for your bodily needs but also supporting your emotional and mental health.

Celebrate the gift of nutrition and self-care with each meal. Accept a broad range of unprocessed, nutrient-rich meals that give your body life. Enjoy the benefits of the occasional indulgence you give yourself guilt-free.

Dear readers, keep in mind that your relationship with food is not a conflict that can be won or lost when you start your Weigh-Down journey. It is a graceful dance that honors self-love, pleasure, and sustenance. Allow this dance to be your compass, pointing you in the direction of freedom and happiness, where food is your ally and guilt and constraint are just distant memories.

Role of self-care activities and stress management in maintaining a positive mindset.

Self-care practices and stress management are crucial to keeping a good outlook while following the Weigh-Down Diet and working towards a healthy weight. Women sometimes find themselves balancing several tasks and demands while being pushed in a million different ways. We must understand that self-care is not a luxury but rather a must for our wellbeing.

Self-care activities help us to refuel and re-establish a stronger connection with ourselves. It may be as easy as taking a soothing bath, doing some meditation, or engaging in an enjoyable pastime. These activities refuel us, ease our tension, and aid in our ability to concentrate and think clearly.

On this road, stress management is equally important. Stress has an influence on our physical health as well as our mental and emotional wellbeing. We may lessen the damaging effects of stress on our bodies by using stress management practices like deep breathing exercises, writing, or seeking help via therapy or counseling.

An optimistic outlook is essential for long-term success. Self-compassion, resilience, and a feeling of balance may all be developed through stress management and self-care. They enable us to overcome obstacles with elegance and flexibility, keeping us from developing self-destructive habits or emotional eating.

In essence, putting self-care first and finding productive ways to deal with stress become pillars of our path. By investing time and energy in these crucial areas, we lay the groundwork for long-term weight reduction, enhanced general wellbeing, and the capacity to live the joyful, meaningful lives we are entitled to.

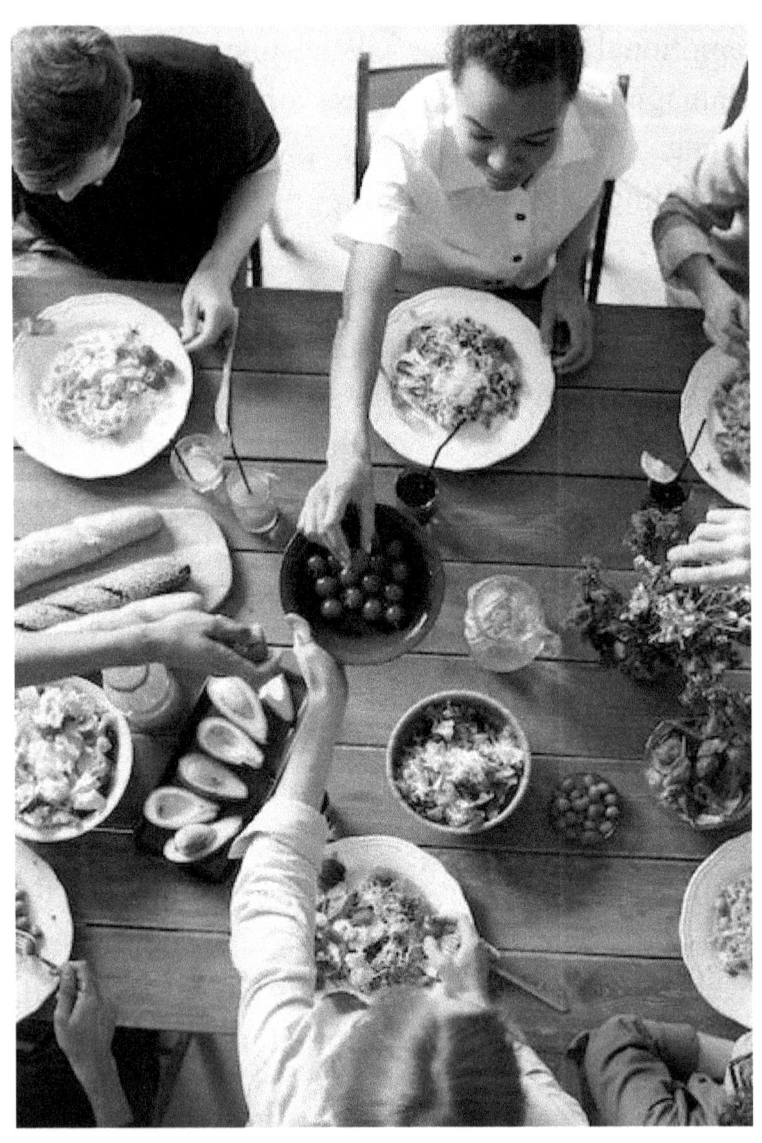

Chapter V

The Power of Movement

The importance of activity cannot be overstated in the quest for a healthy weight and general wellbeing. Exercise has the amazing power to change not only our bodies but also our brains and souls.

Regular exercise not only helps us lose weight and burn calories, but it also improves our mood, gives us more energy, and reduces stress. The ability to move may energize us, activate our senses, and generate endorphins that foster feelings of success and pleasure.

There are various ways to include exercise in our everyday lives, from brisk walks in the outdoors to energizing dancing lessons. We may make exercise enjoyable rather than a chore by engaging in things that we really like. This mental transformation fosters a tenacious and enduring dedication to an active way of life.

Movement also enables us to become aware of our bodies' amazing capacities. We are aware of their fortitude, adaptability, and strength. It gives us the ability to push ourselves, make new resolutions, and go above our own expectations. Every stride, every stretch, and every motion serves as a symbol of our inner fortitude and will.

Movement becomes more than simply a technique to burn calories throughout the weight-Down Diet journey; it becomes a way to celebrate and take care of our bodies. It serves as a reminder that our capacity to move, explore, and fully experience life, rather than the numbers on a scale, defines who we are.

So let's embrace the movement's power, dear reader. Let's move, run, stretch, and fly together. Enjoying physical exercise may change our bodies, thoughts, and spirits, so let's embrace it with delight. We may access a world of bright health, unlimited vitality, and endless possibilities by introducing movement into our daily lives.

The importance of regular physical activity in weight management

Regular physical activity serves as a vital pillar in the field of weight control, especially within the framework of the weight-Down Diet. The route to obtaining and maintaining a healthy weight is multi-faceted, and integrating a regular fitness plan is a critical component of this holistic approach.

First and foremost, participating in regular physical activity considerably contributes to the establishment of a calorie deficit, a key element in weight reduction. Calories expended by physical exercise, when exceeded by the calories ingested, result in weight reduction. This becomes a successful method when paired with attentive, portion-controlled eating encouraged by the Weigh-Down Diet. Physical activity, whether it be aerobic workouts, weight training, or even regular activities like walking, boosts the metabolism, assisting in the effective use of calories and fat for energy.

Furthermore, physical exercise assists in retaining lean muscle mass while decreasing weight. This is significant because muscle tissue demands more energy at rest compared to fat tissue. Hence, the more muscle mass a person has, the greater their resting metabolic rate, boosting weight maintenance after the desired weight is attained.

Exercise also has a key role in controlling stress and boosting mental well-being, qualities frequently disregarded in weight management. Stress may lead to emotional eating or bad dietary choices. Regular physical exercise combats this by generating endorphins, the body's natural mood elevators. It helps relieve anxiety and sadness, encouraging a more balanced attitude toward eating and, subsequently, weight control.

Moreover, exercise favorably benefits general health, lowering the risk of several chronic illnesses, such as heart disease, type 2 diabetes, and some malignancies. In the context of the Weigh-Down Diet, adopting an active lifestyle complements the holistic concept of the program, aiming not just for weight reduction but also for enhanced general health and lifespan.

Caloric Expenditure and Weight Loss:

Engaging in physical exercise expends calories, a key aspect of any weight reduction quest. When the calories burned via exercise exceed the calories ingested from meals, the body draws on stored fat for energy. In combination with the concepts of portion management and mindful eating promoted by the Weigh-Down Diet, regular exercise increases progress towards weight reduction objectives.

Metabolism and Lean Muscle Preservation:

Physical exercise raises the body's metabolism, the rate at which it burns calories during rest. By improving muscle mass and strength through exercise, people maintain and increase lean muscle. Muscles are metabolically active tissues that demand more energy, therefore boosting the basal metabolic rate. This not only assists in weight reduction but also helps maintain weight after the target goal is attained.

Stress management and emotional well-being:

Stress might also additionally cause emotional eating, derailing weight loss attempts. Regular exercise, however, functions as a potent stress reducer. It boosts the creation of endorphins, neurotransmitters that function as natural mood boosters, lowering stress, anxiety, and sadness. By addressing mental well-being, physical exercise fosters better eating behaviors and a more balanced relationship with food, matching the Weigh-Down Diet's holistic approach.

Health Benefits and Disease Prevention:Incorporating exercise into one's lifestyle provides a myriad of health advantages beyond weight control. It promotes cardiovascular health, decreases the risk of chronic illnesses, including type 2 diabetes and heart problems, and boosts bone density. By boosting general health and longevity, frequent physical exercise corresponds with the Weigh-Down Diet's purpose of a holistic, sustainable approach to well-being.

Enhanced energy levels and productivity:

Contrary to a frequent assumption, exercise raises energy levels and combats weariness. Regular physical exercise boosts circulation and increases oxygen flow to cells, boosting vitality and general productivity. This rejuvenated vitality aids people in sustaining an active lifestyle, prolonging the positive cycle of exercise, and making well-informed nutritional choices encouraged by the Weigh-Down Diet. Community and Support:

Incorporating physical exercise typically includes participating in a community, whether in a gym, a fitness class, or outdoor activities. This feeling of community generates support, motivation, and a sense of belonging—vital aspects in sustaining a regular exercise program and sticking to the principles of the Weigh-Down Diet in the long run.

Types of exercises suitable for women and suggestions to incorporate women into daily routines

Exercise is an essential component of any successful weight control regimen, including the Weigh-Down Diet. For women, choosing an exercise regimen that matches their lifestyle and interests is crucial to consistency and long-term success. Here are numerous sorts of workouts ideal for women, along with advice on how to include them in everyday routines:

Cardiovascular Exercises:
Types: Walking, jogging, running, cycling, swimming, dancing, and aerobics.
Incorporation: Start with a daily brisk walk or a bike ride in your neighborhood. Opt for activities you like to make it a regular habit.

Strength Training:

Types: bodyweight exercises (e.g., push-ups, squats, lunges), weight lifting, resistance band exercises, and utilizing gym equipment.

Incorporation: Incorporate bodyweight workouts during breaks or during cooking. Consider a 30-minute strength training session 2-3 times a week.

Yoga and Pilates:

Types: Hatha, Vinyasa, Ashtanga, and Power Yoga; Pilates workouts for core strength and flexibility.

Incorporation: Begin your day with a quick yoga or Pilates program. Use internet videos or applications for guided sessions.

High-Intensity Interval Training (HIIT):

Types: quick, intense bursts of activity followed by intervals of relaxation.

Incorporation: Dedicate 20-30 minutes, 2-3 times a week, for an HIIT exercise. This may be done at home with no equipment.

Group Classes:

Types: Zumba, spinning, step aerobics, and group fitness courses in gyms or studios.

Incorporation: Join a local fitness class that matches your schedule and preferences, whether it's before or after work.

Flexibility and Mobility Exercises:

Types: Stretching, mobility exercises, Tai Chi.

Incorporation: Stretch while watching TV or include a few stretches into your daily routine to increase flexibility.

Outdoor Activities:

Types: Hiking, running in the park, outdoor cycling, kayaking, and paddleboarding.

Incorporation: Plan weekend outside activities that incorporate exercise and fresh air.

Mind-Body Exercises:

Types: Tai Chi, Qigong, mindfulness-based stress reduction (MBSR), and deep breathing techniques.

Incorporation: Incorporate mindfulness and relaxation practices into your everyday routine, even if it's only for a few minutes.

Barre Workouts:

Benefits: Improves strength, flexibility, and posture with a blend of ballet-inspired motions and isometric holds.

Incorporation: Follow online barre fitness sessions at home. Use a strong chair or countertop as a support for balance.

Aqua Aerobics:

Benefits: Low-impact workout that's mild on the joints while providing resistance to increase muscular tone and cardiovascular conditioning.

Incorporation: Join a local water aerobics class at a nearby pool. Aim for 2-3 workouts each week for optimum results.

Circuit Training:

Benefits: It combines strength and aerobic training, boosting overall fitness and calorie burn.

Incorporation: Create a circuit program using bodyweight exercises (e.g., push-ups, squats, burpees) and do each activity for a minute, resting in between. Repeat for 3-4 cycles.

Dance Workouts:

Benefits: A delightful approach to enhancing cardiovascular fitness, coordination, and mental well-being.

Incorporation: Put on your favorite music and dance about the home. Consider taking dancing lessons or utilizing online dance fitness courses.

Martial Arts:

Benefits: Enhances self-defense abilities, balance, flexibility, and strength.

Incorporation: Enroll in a local martial arts class or study training DVDs for novices at home.

Stability Ball Workouts:

Benefits: It builds core strength, improves balance, and utilizes muscles that may not be recruited during normal activities.

Incorporation: Swap your workplace chair with a stability ball to exercise your core while working. Incorporate stability ball workouts with your strength training regimen.

Rebounding:

Benefits: A pleasant and low-impact aerobic exercise that improves balance, coordination, and lymphatic circulation.

Incorporation: Invest in a rebounder (mini-trampoline) and rebound while watching TV or during breaks.

Benefits of staying active beyond weight loss include improved mood, increased energy, and overall well-being.

In the domain of the Weigh-Down Diet, the path towards a healthy weight is merely one part of the greater tapestry created by an active lifestyle. Physical exercise, although crucial in accomplishing weight control objectives, extends its reach well beyond the bounds of a scale. It evolves into a portal towards comprehensive well-being, enhancing life with a range of magnificent advantages that stretch to the very center of our existence.

1. Enhanced mood and mental clarity:

Physical exercise causes the production of endorphins, the body's natural mood boosters. Engaging in regular exercise cultivates a deep feeling of well-being and considerably alleviates stress, anxiety, and sadness. The rush of endorphins causes a euphoric mood, frequently referred to as a "runner's high," that may be equivalent to a medicinal elixir for the mind.

2. Amplified Energy Levels:

Contrary to the perception that effort depletes energy, physical exercise is a significant catalyst for improving overall energy levels. Regular exercise increases cardiovascular health, leading to enhanced circulation and higher stamina. As the body becomes more effective at using oxygen and nutrients, ordinary chores become less exhausting, leaving you feeling energized and ready to confront the day.

3. Heightened Cognitive Function:

Exercise not only fortifies muscles but also sharpens the intellect. Regular physical exercise is associated with increased cognitive performance, including greater memory, attention, and creativity. It encourages the creation of new neurons and improves the connections between existing ones, a process known as neuroplasticity. As a consequence, an active lifestyle is connected with a sharper mind and a more robust brain.

4. Quality sleep and relaxation:

A balanced exercise plan promotes improved sleep by regulating circadian rhythms and boosting sleep quality. Restorative sleep, in turn, boosts mood, cognitive function, and general mental sharpness. Physical exercise functions as a natural sedative, helping you fall asleep sooner and experience deeper, more restful slumber.

5. Longevity and Healthspan Extension:

Regular physical exercise is a cornerstone of a healthy lifespan. Engaging in exercise improves your lifetime by lowering the risk of chronic illnesses such as cardiovascular disease, diabetes, and some malignancies. Additionally, keeping active extends your healthspan—the number of years you live in excellent health—enabling you to enjoy a robust, satisfying life as you age.

6. Self-confidence and Self-Esteem:

Physical exercise cultivates a good body image and encourages self-acceptance. Achieving exercise objectives, no matter how minor, feeds a feeling of success and promotes self-esteem.

The empowerment that develops from surmounting physical obstacles transcends the gym, impacting how you view and conduct yourself in other facets of life.

7. Strengthened Immune System:

Regular physical exercise is a cornerstone of a healthy immune system. Exercise helps flush out toxins from the body via sweating and promotes healthier lymphatic circulation. It also promotes the formation of white blood cells, which are crucial for fighting off infections and disorders. By remaining active, you boost your body's defensive systems and lower the danger of being ill.

8. Enhanced Social Interaction and Community Building:

Engaging in group workouts, sports, or even solitary physical activities in public settings generally leads to improved social contact. Whether it's a friendly game of basketball, a yoga session, or a jog in the park, these activities provide chances to interact with like-minded others. Socializing while exercising may ease feelings of loneliness, boost motivation, and create a sense of connection and community.

9. Improved Posture and Flexibility:

Regular physical activity, especially workouts that concentrate on strength and flexibility, helps to improve posture. Stronger muscles in the core, back, and shoulders support the spine and promote an upright posture. Moreover, flexibility activities like yoga and stretching promote joint mobility and lower the risk of accidents, allowing for a more agile and pleasant everyday life.

10. Better Heart Health and Circulation:

Exercise is a tonic for the heart and circulatory system. It assists in decreasing bad cholesterol (LDL) and boosting good cholesterol (HDL), resulting in a healthier heart. Regular physical exercise lowers blood pressure, reduces the danger of plaque development in arteries, and minimizes the possibility of heart disease. By encouraging excellent heart health, exercise guarantees a longer, more active life.

11. Relaxation and stress reduction:

Engaging in physical exercise functions as an effective stress reducer. Exercise aids in reducing cortisol levels, the hormone linked with stress, and causes the production of endorphins, which generate a sensation of calm. It gives a healthy outlet for handling life's demands, encouraging mental clarity and emotional balance.

Chapter VI

Overcoming Challenges and Staying Motivated

The Nature of Challenges

Understanding the nature of obstacles is the first step towards conquering them. Challenges may arise in numerous forms—emotional, physical, social, or situational. Emotional troubles may also consist of stress, emotional eating, or a terrible self-image. Physical obstacles involve health concerns, exhaustion, or plateaus in weight reduction. Cultural issues sometimes originate from cultural pressures and body image standards. Circumstantial problems encompass time limits, a lack of resources, or lifestyle adjustments.

Attentionals to Overcome Challenges

attentive Awareness: The cornerstone of overcoming problems resides in attentive awareness. Recognize and embrace the challenge without judgment. Understand its nature and accept its influence on your trip. By admitting the difficulty, you empower yourself to discover a solution.

Adaptability: Embrace adaptability as an important characteristic. Flexibility in your approach allows for modifications as issues arise. If a certain component of the diet isn't working for you, be open to adjusting it to fit your circumstances while still complying with the diet's main ideals.

Seek Support: You're not alone on this path. Reach out to a support network, whether it is a friend, a support group, or a healthcare professional. Sharing your concerns and getting assistance might bring fresh views and revive motivation.

Goal Refinement: Revisit and revise your objectives. Break them into tiny, manageable goals. Celebrate your progress, irrespective of how tiny. This reinforcement builds motivation and keeps you on track.

Self-Compassion and Patience: Be kind with yourself. Understand that development takes time, and failures are a normal part of any journey. Practice self-compassion, forgive yourself for slip-ups, and continue with fresh drive.

Sustaining Motivation

Visualization and Affirmations: Envision your eventual aim. Create a mental picture of your better, fitter self. Use affirmations to strengthen your commitment. The more clearly you can visualize your accomplishment, the more real and achievable it becomes.

Positive Reinforcement: Surround yourself with optimism. Engage with success stories, motivating books or inspirational role models. Let their stories inspire your own drive and boost your dedication to the Weigh-Down Diet.

Regular Reflection: Set aside time periodically to reflect on your progress. Celebrate your achievements and assess your problems. Understand how far you've come and how much closer you are to your objective. This reflection reignites drive.

Incorporate range: Keep the diet fresh and enjoyable by adding a range of nutritious foods and unique dishes. Mundanity may inhibit drive, so embrace variation in your food planning to make the trip intriguing.

Common obstacles faced during weight loss journeys and strategies for overcoming them

As someone passionately involved in the areas of health and wellness, I've seen countless ladies on their weight reduction journeys. Each trip is as unique as the person pursuing it, yet similar barriers typically arise. Recognizing and resolving these challenges is key to sustained growth and enduring success on the Weigh-Down Diet.

Emotional Eating with Stress:

Obstacle: Emotional ingesting might also additionally undermine the fine of intentions. Stress, worry, depression, or even pleasure may induce a desire to eat, frequently leading to poor decisions.

Strategy: Implement thoughtful techniques like deep breathing, meditation, or journaling to manage stress. Channel emotional reactions into non-food-related activities like exercise, drawing, or spending time with loved ones.

Unrealistic Expectations:

Obstacle: Unrealistic ambitions may lead to irritation and disappointment, forcing some to stop their efforts early.

Strategy: Set manageable, progressive objectives. Celebrate minor accomplishments along the way and remember that lasting weight reduction takes time.

Lack of Time for Meal Preparation:

Obstacle: Busy schedules may make it tough to prepare healthy meals, frequently leading to reverting to fast food or unhealthy snacks.

Strategy: Plan meals in advance, batch-cook on weekends, or go for fast, nutritious options like smoothies, salads, or pre-cut vegetables with hummus.

Social Pressure and Environments:

Obstacle: Social gatherings and office cultures may not always fit with a healthy eating plan, making it tough to remain on track.

Strategy: Communicate your goals to close friends and coworkers, asking for their support. Prepare for social engagements by having a healthy snack beforehand or volunteering to bring food that corresponds with your dietary preferences.

Plateaus and Slow Progress:

Obstacle: Weight reduction plateaus may be depressing, making it tough to remain motivated.

Strategy: Mix up your routine - adjust your exercise, try different dishes, or see a dietician for modifications. Focus on non-scale achievements, like higher energy or better sleep.

Cravings for Unhealthy Foods:

Obstacle: Cravings for unhealthy meals may hinder progress and derail the best-laid efforts.

Strategy: Find healthy alternatives for your desires and exercise portion control. Engage in activities like walking, reading, or hobbies to distract your thoughts from your desires.

Self-Image and Body Confidence:

Obstacle: Negative self-image may hamper growth and lead to cycles of harmful habits.

Strategy: Practice self-compassion and surround yourself with good influences. Seek assistance from a mental health professional if body image concerns continue.

Lack of consistency:

Obstacle: Inconsistency in food and exercise routines might hamper growth and inhibit the establishment of durable habits.

Strategy: Establish a regimen and adhere to it as closely as possible. Prioritize consistency above intensity, even if it means beginning with tiny, doable improvements. Gradually build upon these adjustments for permanent outcomes.

Nutritional Misinformation:

Obstacle: The plethora of contradictory nutritional information may be confusing and may lead to inappropriate eating choices.

Strategy: Rely on credible sources for dietary recommendations, and see a qualified dietitian if required. Focus on complete, unprocessed foods and stress a balanced diet with a range of nutrients.

Lack of support system:

Obstacle: Attempting to reduce weight alone without a support system may be alienating and demotivating.

Strategy: Surround yourself with a supporting network—whether it's a friend, family member, or an online group. Having someone to discuss your struggles, efforts, and triumphs may bring encouragement and accountability.

Physical Limitations or Health Issues:

Obstacle: Existing health issues or physical restrictions may hinder some workouts or food choices.

Strategy: Consult a healthcare expert before beginning any diet or activity regimen. They may give customized advice and safe alternatives to fit your individual health demands and situations.

Overwhelming Information Overload:

Obstacle: The large quantity of weight reduction information accessible may be intimidating, making it difficult to select the optimal technique.

Strategy: Simplify your approach by concentrating on key concepts of the Weigh-Down Diet: intuitive eating, mindful feeding, and gradual, lasting improvements. Trust the process and avoid becoming bogged down by abundant, contradicting information.

Financial Constraints:

Obstacle: A sense that eating well is costly might dissuade people from making better choices.

Strategy: Plan budget-friendly meals utilizing cost-effective, nutrient-dense foods including grains, legumes, seasonal vegetables, and bulk products. Look for deals, coupons, and local markets for inexpensive solutions.

Binge Eating and Food Addiction:

Obstacle: Overcoming tendencies toward binge eating or food addiction takes specific tactics and help.

Strategy: Seek help from a mental health professional or support group specializing in eating problems. Cognitive-behavioral therapy (CBT) and mindfulness practices may be effective aids in addressing and overcoming these issues.

Tips for managing cravings, dealing with social situations, and staying motivated in the face of setbacks

Navigating the weight-Down Diet involves not just a dedication to healthy food but also the grit to control cravings, navigate social settings, and overcome disappointments. Here are some expert recommendations to aid you along this inspiring journey:

Managing Cravings: Mindful Awareness:

Recognize your goals without judgment. Understand the triggers and feelings linked to them. Are you actually hungry, or is it stress, boredom, or habit fueling the craving?

Healthy Substitutions:

Substitute unhealthy appetites with healthy ones. If you desire sweets, go for fruits. If you want something salty, try nuts or seeds. Gradually, your palette will adjust to these healthier options.

Hydration:

Often, thirst may be confused with hunger or desire. Drink water when hunger strikes, and observe if it diminishes. Staying well-hydrated may minimize needless munching.

Plan Ahead:

Have healthy foods readily accessible. Pre-cut fruits, vegetables, or a handful of almonds may be filling, so avoid impulsive, harmful choices.

Dealing with social situations:

Communicate Your Goals: When attending social events, explain your dietary goals appropriately. Friends and relatives frequently appreciate and support your efforts if they understand your aims.

Volunteer to contribute:

If suitable, volunteer to bring food that corresponds with your nutritional objectives. This ensures you have a healthy choice accessible and also exposes others to nutritional options.

Emphasis on company, not just food:

Shift the emphasis of social events from the food to the company and discussions. Engage in talks, games, or activities that shift the focus away from eating.

Practice Saying No:

It's alright to respectfully refuse offers of food or drink that don't correspond with your objectives. Practice saying no assertively but gracefully.

Staying Motivated in the Face of Setbacks:

Forgive Yourself: Understand that setbacks are a normal part of every endeavor. Forgive yourself and utilize failures as learning opportunities, not excuses to quit.

Set SMART objectives:

Specific, Measurable, Achievable, Relevant, and Time-bound objectives keep you focused and motivated. Celebrate your successes, irrespective of how minor.

Seek support and Accountability:

Share your journey with a supportive friend, join a support group, or seek a professional nutritionist. Having someone to discuss your struggles and successes with may enhance motivation.

Visualize Success:

Imagine yourself reaching your objective and enjoying enhanced health and confidence. Use this graphic to spark your drive while experiencing setbacks.

The importance of self-compassion and the celebration of non-scale victories

On the road towards a healthy and balanced life with the Weigh-Down Diet, one frequently forgotten but vital part is the practice of self-compassion and the celebration of non-scale triumphs.

The process of obtaining and maintaining a healthy weight is more than simply numbers on a scale—it's about building a good connection with oneself and recognizing success beyond just weight reduction.

Self-compassion is the skill of treating oneself with the same love, care, and understanding that we would provide a close friend. When seeking weight control, it's vital to exercise self-compassion during the ups and downs of the path. This means appreciating our efforts, embracing shortcomings, and forgiving ourselves for any failures.

It's about realizing that perfection is not the objective, but development is.

By practicing self-compassion, we build a caring atmosphere inside ourselves. We learn to love our bodies as they are, understanding that they're always growing. This mentality adjustment helps to lessen the tension and worry commonly connected with the dieting process. Instead of self-criticism, we fill our path with love and support, motivating us to persist even when confronted with hardships.

Equally crucial is recognizing non-scale wins, which reach beyond the numbers displayed on a scale. Non-scale successes cover different milestones on the way to a healthy lifestyle: an increase in energy levels, better sleep habits, greater mental clarity, heightened self-confidence, or the capacity to handle stress more efficiently. These successes are a credit to our hard work, devotion, and perseverance.

Celebrating non-scale accomplishments helps change the emphasis from a limited view of success to a comprehensive viewpoint of well-being. It urges us to realize the transforming influence of the Weigh-Down diet on our entire quality of life. Whether it's being able to finish an exercise regimen, fitting into a smaller clothing size, or getting comments on our healthy glow, these wins encourage and strengthen our dedication to the path.

Moreover, self-compassion builds resilience. It works as a shield against the negativity that might hinder growth. In periods of hardship, it's the self-compassionate voice that reminds us of how far we've gone, how much we've learned, and that every step, no matter how tiny, is a step forward. This kindness to oneself is not only an emotional balm; it's a driver for development and enduring change.

On the other side, celebrating non-scale triumphs is a discipline founded on gratitude and mindfulness. It moves our emphasis from what the scale prescribes to the huge range of good changes that occur inside ourselves and around us. The vibrant shine of healthy skin, the fortitude to walk up a flight of stairs without gasping, the renewed delight in physical activities—these wins are riches worth celebrating.

These events underscore the concept that health is complex. It's not just about the inches dropped, but the inches gained in self-confidence and self-awareness. It's about valuing the work, devotion, and discipline involved, irrespective of the stats. These non-scale wins are like stepping stones, each one moving us ahead on our transforming path.

In conclusion, self-compassion and the celebration of non-scale triumphs are not merely decorations to the Weigh-Down diet; they are foundations of strength and resilience. They promote a good self-imagedevelop our mental and emotional well-being, and cement our commitment to continue this path with love, joy, and an unflinching conviction in our ability for development and change. Through these activities, we not only gain a healthy physique but also create a genuine, permanent love for ourselves—a love that is the cornerstone of a really satisfying existence.

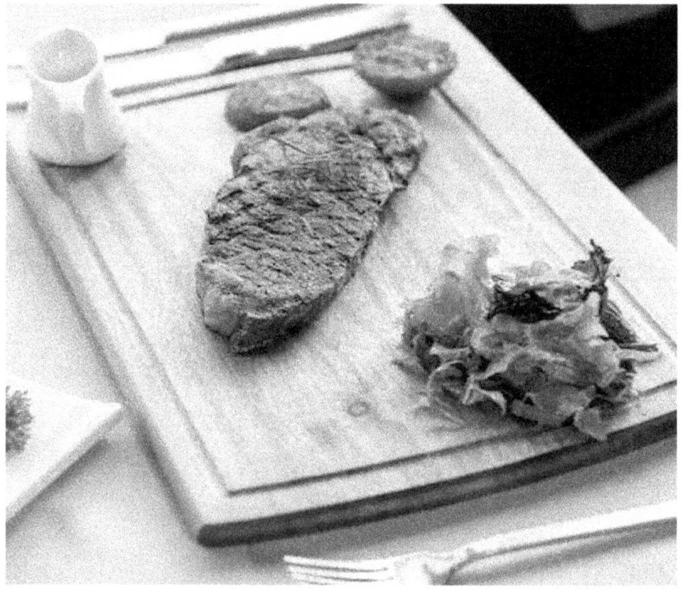

Conclusion

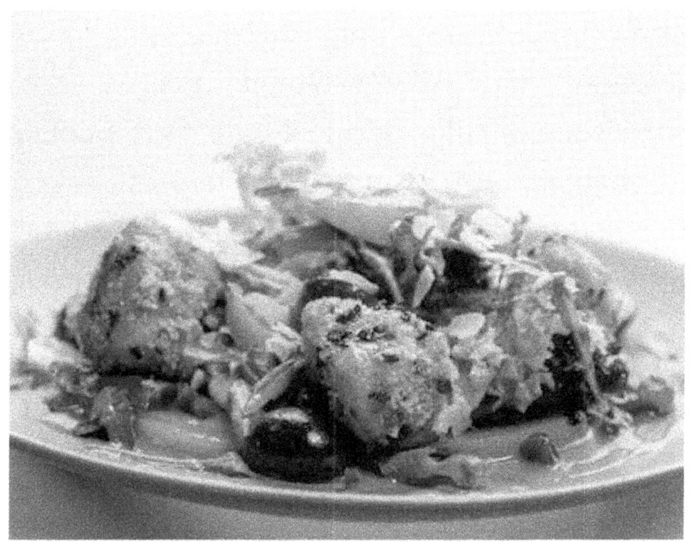

As our adventure through the Weigh-Down Diet for women draws to an end, I am overwhelmed with a feeling of excitement and success. We have examined the depths of self-discovery, the intricacies of our relationships with food, and the transforming force that resides inside us all. It has been an adventure distinguished by drive, perseverance, and the unshakeable optimism that we can indeed choose a lighter, better route for ourselves.

Through the pages of this book, we have demolished the traditional conceptions of dieting, redefining our approach to weight reduction. The Weigh-Down diet is not a rigorous set of rules or a fast cure; it is a concept that enables us to listen to our bodies, to relish the essence of healthy meals, and to celebrate our well-being. It's an encouragement to find balance, not just in our diets but in our lives as a whole.

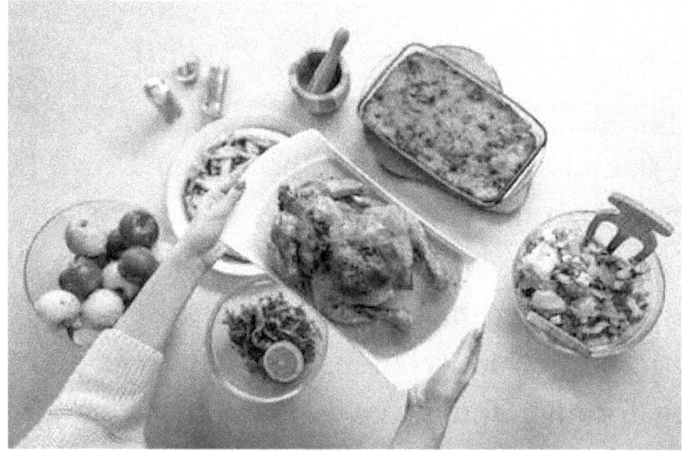

We've understood that genuine health is a combination of the physical, emotional, and spiritual parts of our existence. It's about sustaining ourselves with love, self-compassion, and understanding. It's about understanding when to celebrate our accomplishments and how to learn from our losses without self-condemnation.

In the center of this transforming journey, we rediscovered the deep beauty of intuitive eating—the skill of tuning into our bodies and responding to their needs with love. We learned that hunger is not the enemy but a message pointing us toward nutrition. We found peace in attentive eating, in the ritual of each meal, and in the appreciation of the nutrition that nature offers.

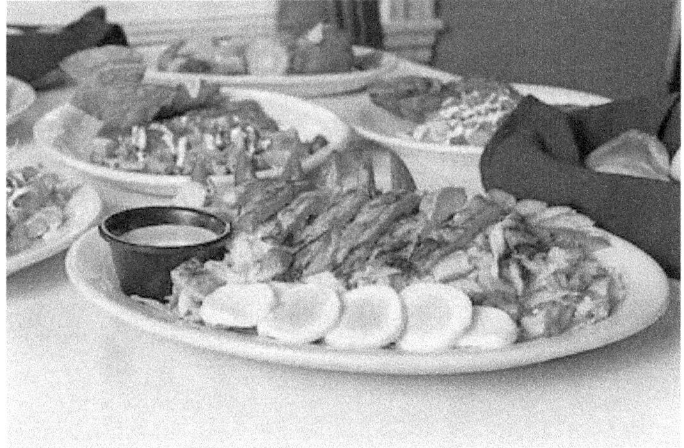

Exercise became more than simply a tool for weight control; it became a celebration of movement, a way to celebrate the wonderful vessel that carries us through life. We embraced diverse types of action, realizing that every stride, every stretch, and every breath is a step towards a better, happier version of ourselves.

And on this voyage, we did not travel alone. We developed a community—a sisterhood of support—sharing our wins and tribulations and pushing each other up. We discovered that our individual tales, although distinct, are fashioned from the same fabric of resolve and hope. Together, we established an atmosphere of support, inspiration, and love—a place where change is not just possible but inevitable.

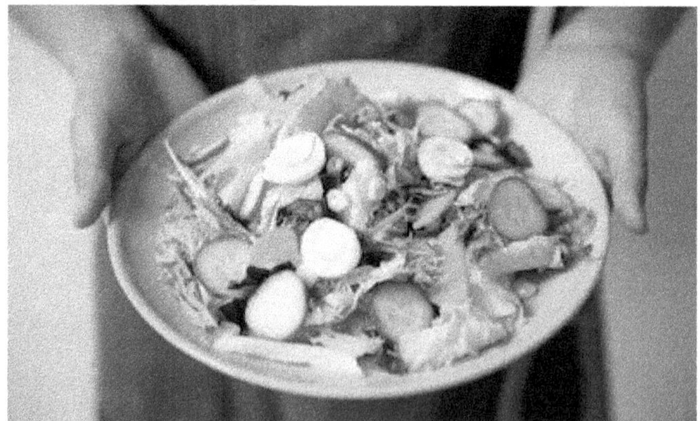

As we say goodbye to this book, I ask you to carry the flame of knowledge and empowerment onward. Let this newfound insight guide your way, and let the Weigh-Down Diet be not just a phase but a lifestyle—a celebration of your strength, perseverance, and love for the wonderful person that is you.

May your journey always be blessed with lightness, love, and the unshakeable trust in your power to select a route that values your body, mind, and soul. You are capable of everything you put your heart and mind to.

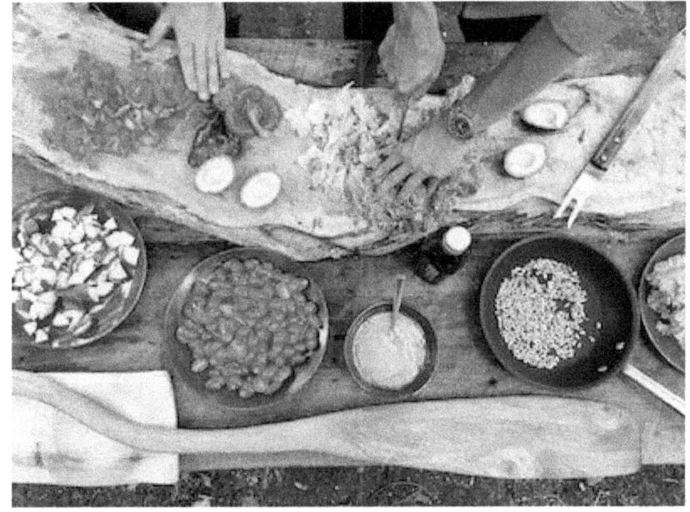

Recap the key principles of the Weigh-Down Diet for women

Intuitive Eating and Mindful Awareness:Listen to your body's hunger and fullness signals.

Eat attentively, paying attention to the flavor, texture, and enjoyment obtained from eating.

Portion Control and Balanced Nutrition:

Be conscious of portion amounts to prevent overeating.

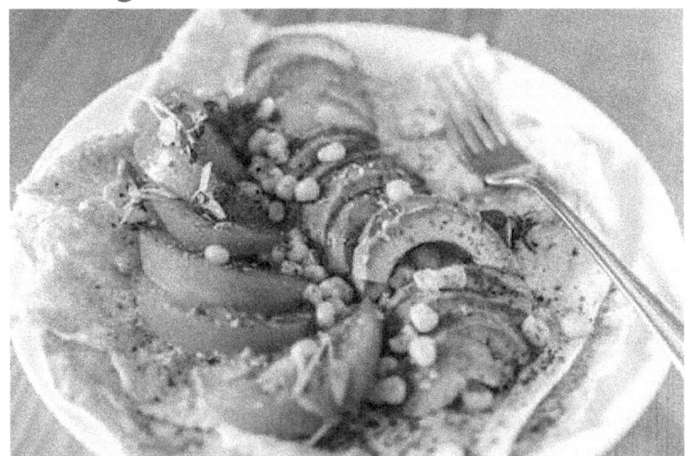

Embrace a balanced diet rich in fruits, vegetables, lean meats, and whole grains.

Emotional Well-Being and Self-Reflection:
Address emotional eating by knowing triggers and establishing appropriate coping techniques. Reflect on your connection with food and build a good perspective.

Physical Activity and Movement:
Incorporate frequent physical exercise into your regimen, suited to your tastes and fitness level.

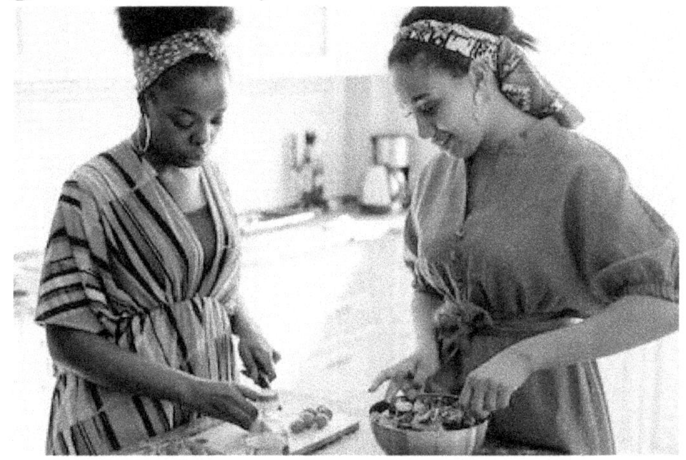

Understand that activity is not just for weight reduction but for complete well-being and energy.

Lifestyle and Sustainable Choices: Strive for long-term, sustainable improvements in your lifestyle rather than fast solutions.

Make modest, realistic improvements to your behaviors for enduring effects.

Community and Support:

Seek and offer support within a community of like-minded folks on a similar path.

Share experiences, problems, and accomplishments to keep motivated and encouraged.

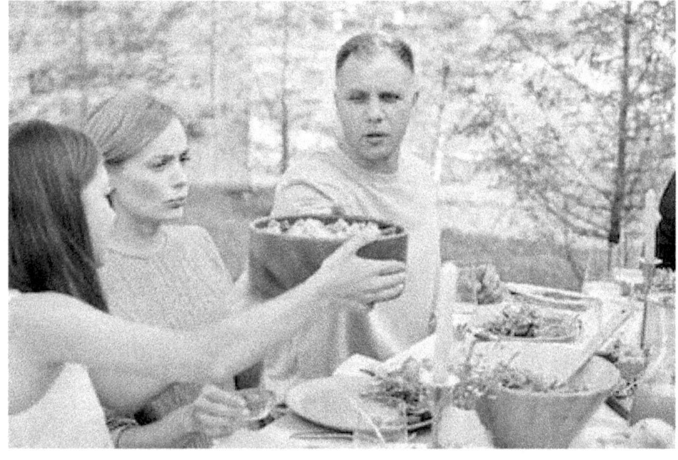

Self-Compassion and Non-Scale Victories:
Practice self-compassion, being compassionate with oneself amid setbacks or perceived failures. Celebrate victories beyond the scale, celebrating improvements in mental, emotional, and physical well-being.

Personalized Approach:
Tailor the Weigh-Down Diet to your own needs, tastes, and health concerns.
Understand that what works for one person may not work precisely the same way for another; accept your own path.

Encouraging readers to embrace a lifelong commitment to their health and well-being

Your health is your lifetime companion. Embrace it, nurture it, and celebrate it. Every decision counts. Choose a route of health because it's a journey that leads to a life of vigor and pleasure. Start now and never look back.

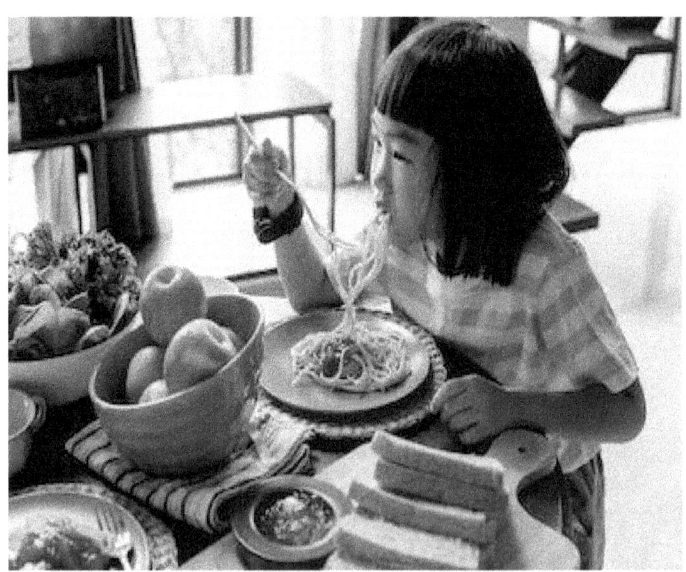

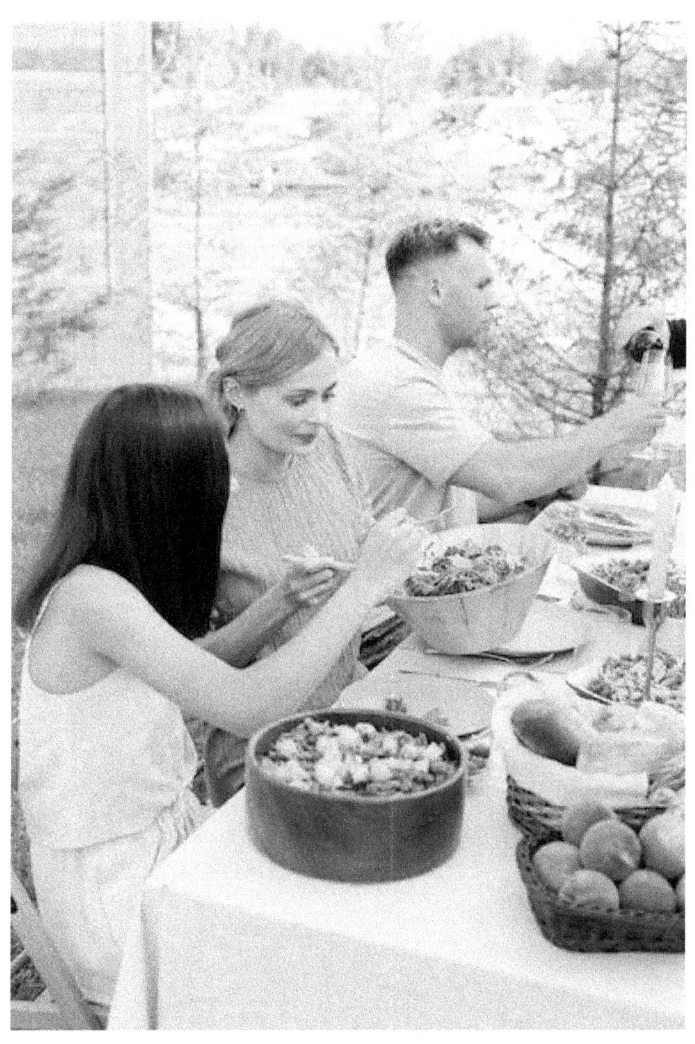

DEAR WOMEN,

Please, if you appreciate this book, consider giving it a favorable review, I hope this message finds you well. I'm reaching out to humbly seek your honest evaluation of my book.

*A positive review from one of our honest customers like you makes others feel secure about selecting **"The Complete Weigh Down Diet For Women"**, Sharing your joyful experience will be much welcomed and push me to write more books for your happiness.*

Your review will assist prospective readers and influence their expectations. Your thoughts will be the reason someone chooses to plunge into this literary experience. I'd greatly appreciate your sincere input.

Thanks *for considering this request.*
Best regards.

Meal planner
Week 1

Weekly meal plan journal

Date: ______________

Monday

Breakfast

Lunch

Dinner

Snacks

Tuesday

Breakfast

Lunch

Dinner

Snacks

Wednesday

Breakfast

Lunch

Dinner

Snacks

Thursday

Breakfast

Lunch

Dinner

Snacks

Friday

Breakfast

Lunch

Dinner

Snacks

Saturday

Breakfast

Lunch

Dinner

Snacks

Sunday

Breakfast

Lunch

Dinner

Snacks

Notes

The Complete Weigh Down Diet For Women

Meal plan week 2

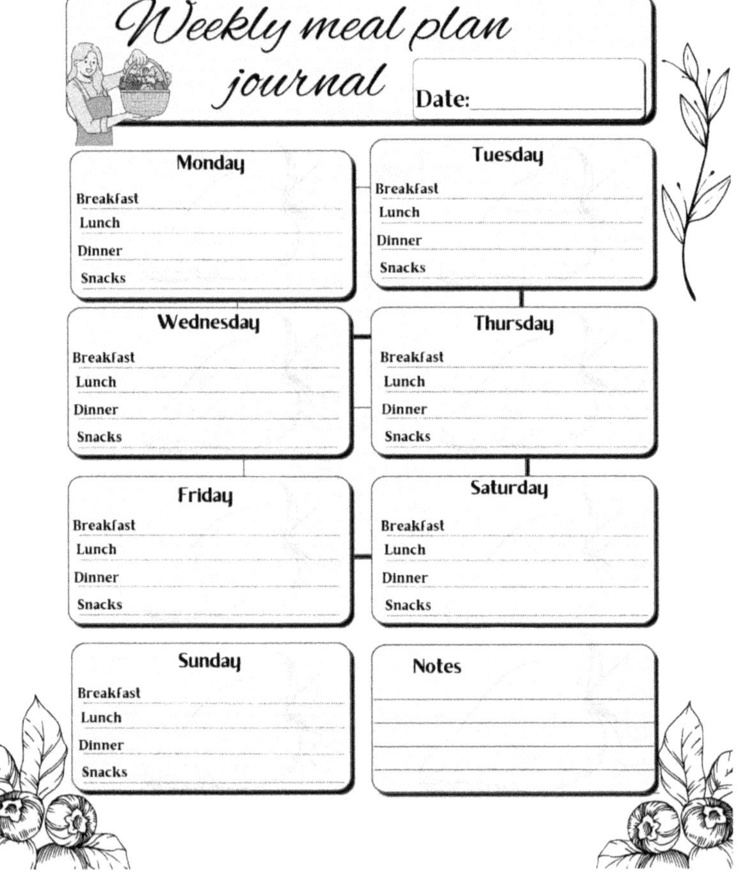

Meal plan week 3

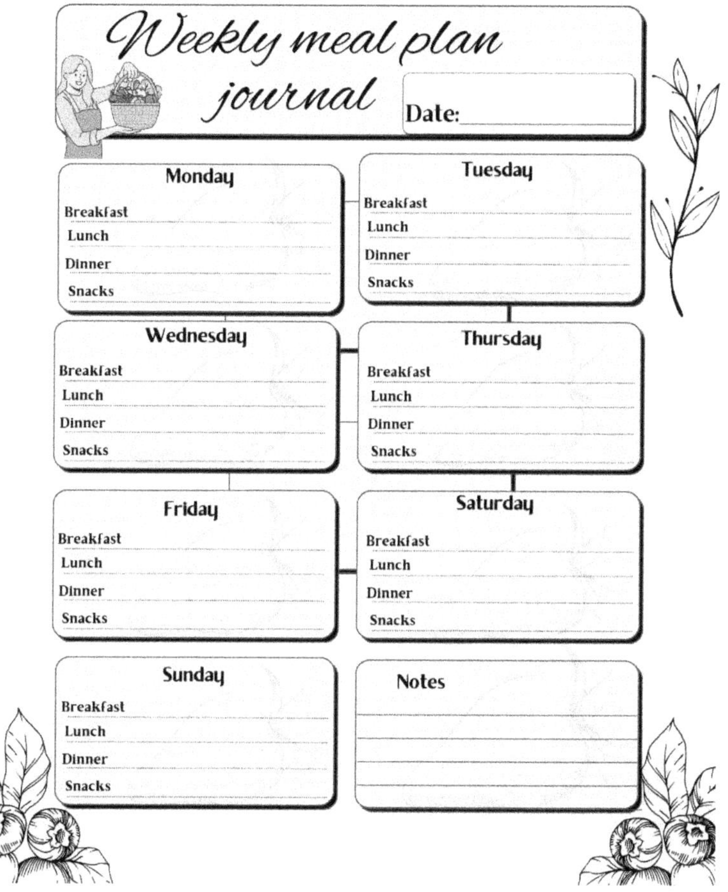

The Complete Weigh Down Diet For Women

Meal plan week 4

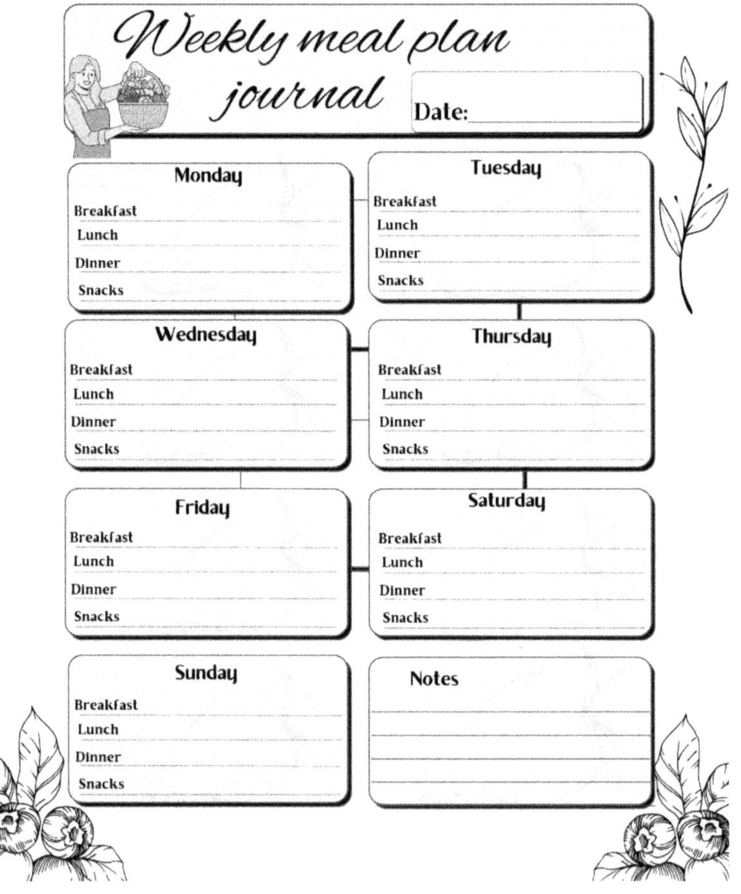

The Complete Weigh Down Diet For Women

Meal plan week 5

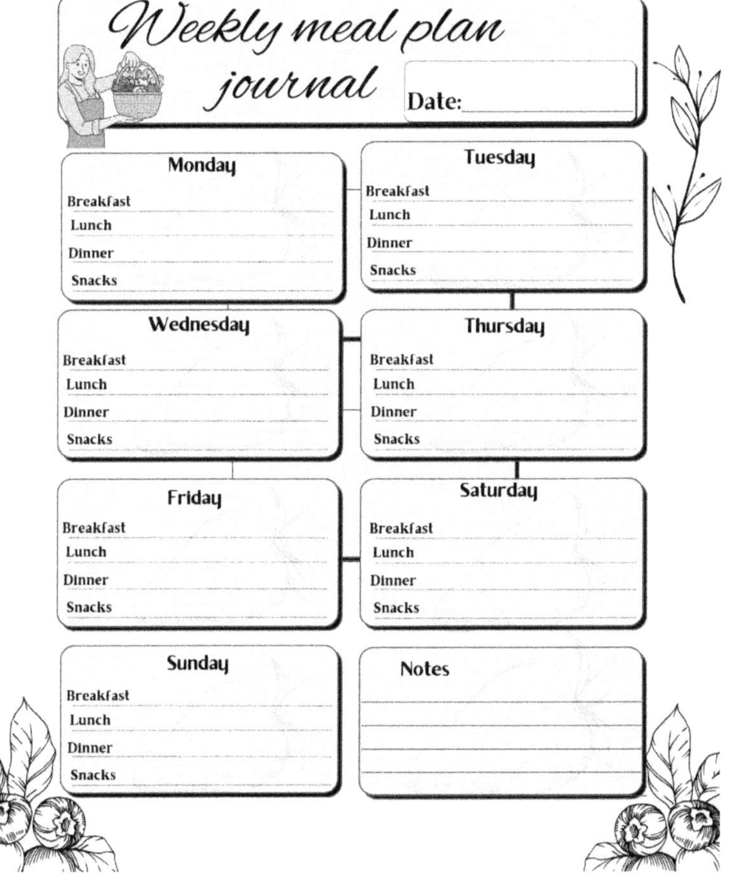

Meal plan week 6

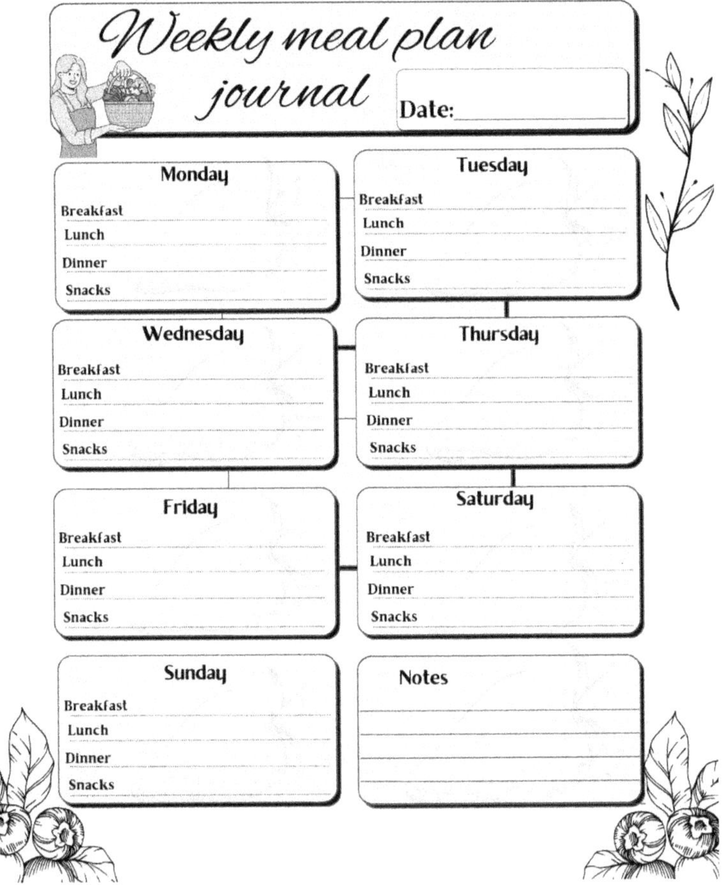

Meal plan week 7

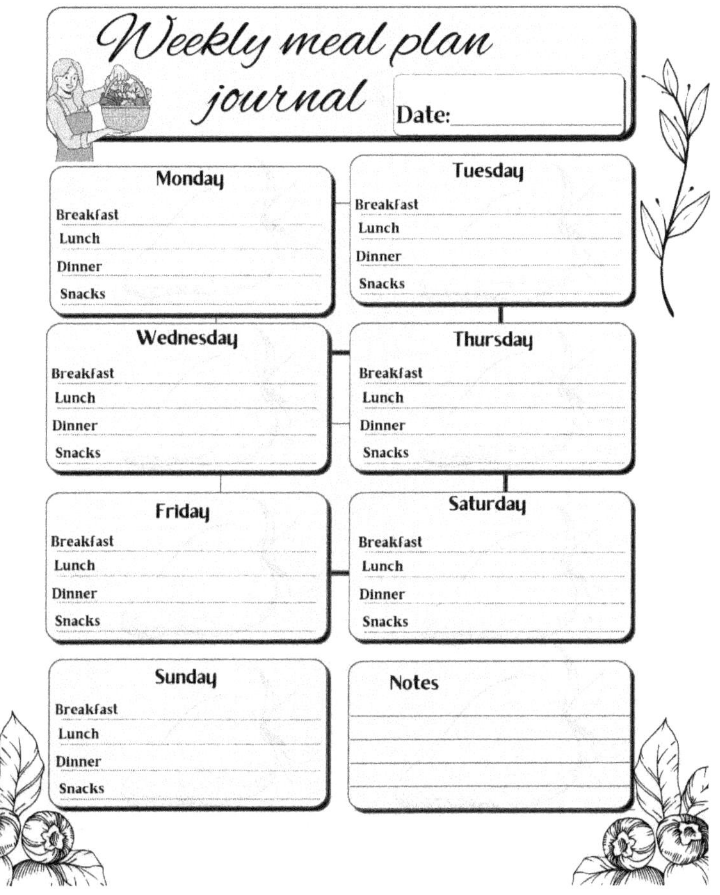

Meal plan week 8

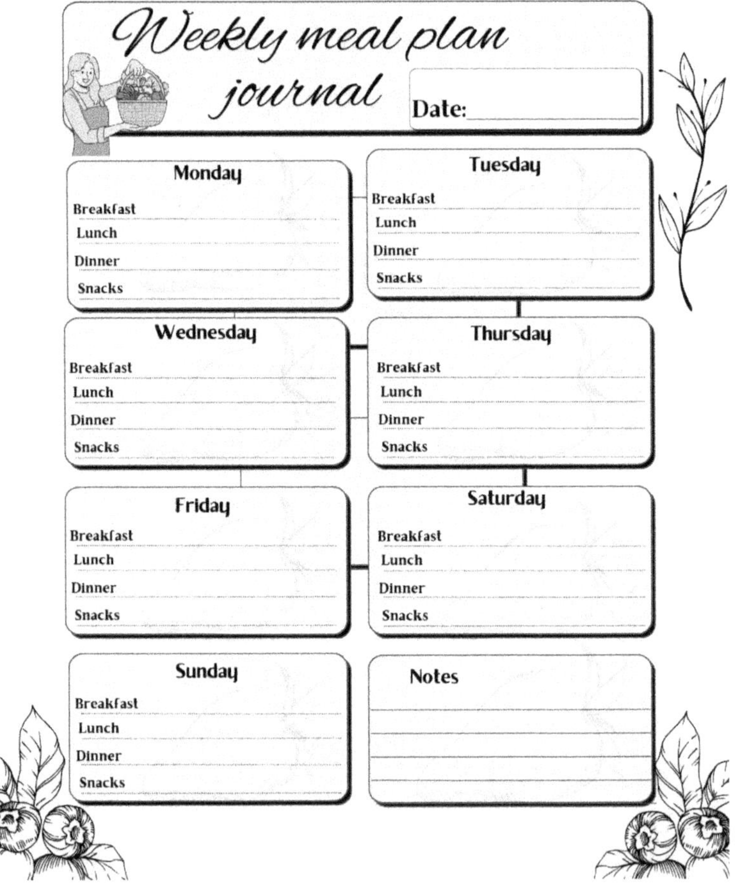

Meal plan week 9

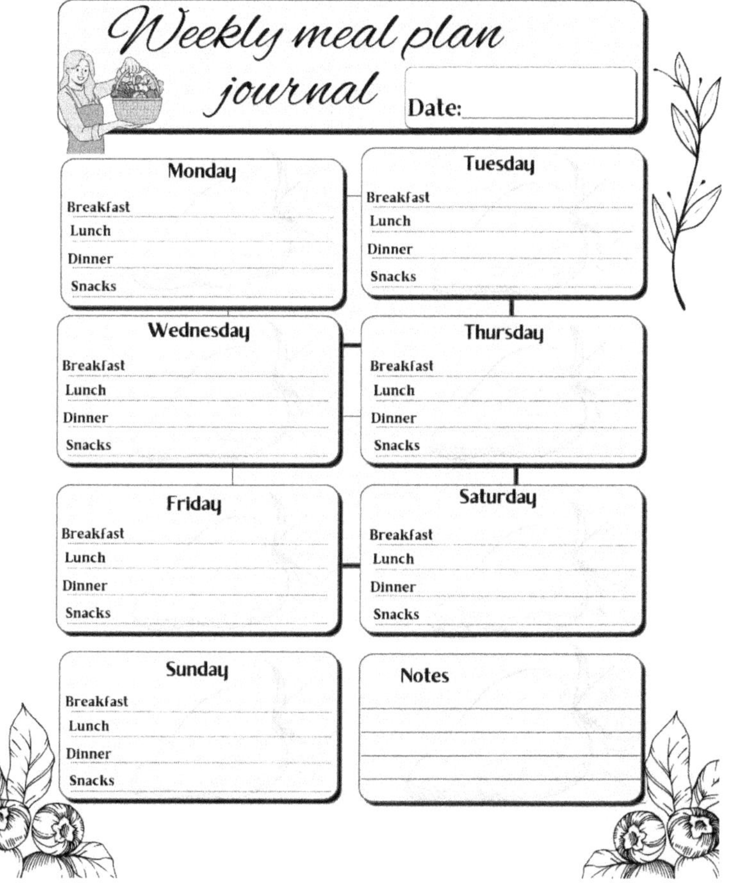

The Complete Weigh Down Diet For Women

Meal plan week 10

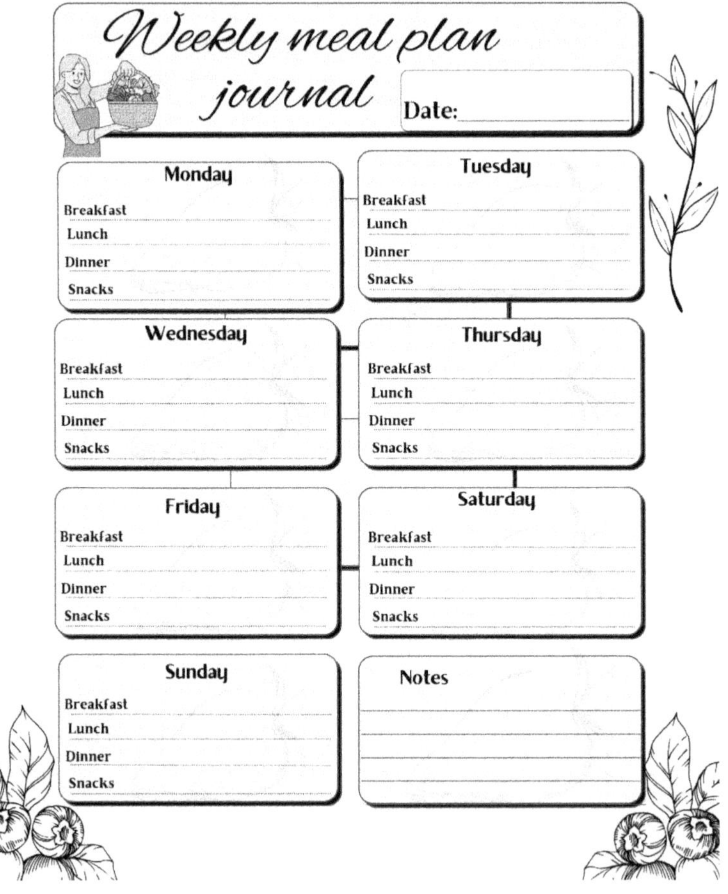

The Complete Weigh Down Diet For Women

Meal plan week 11

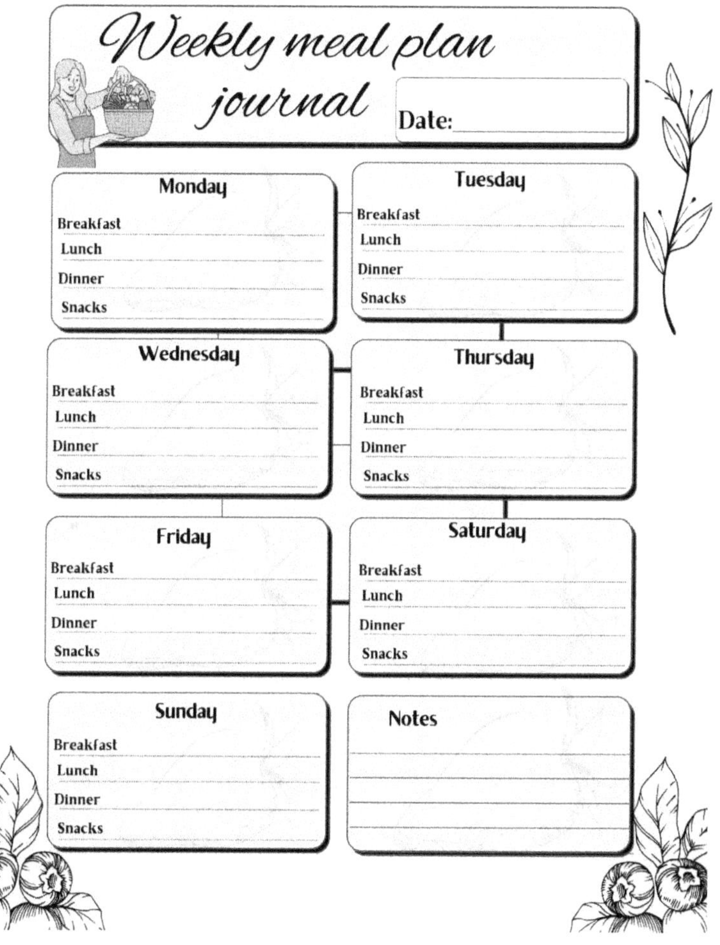

The Complete Weigh Down Diet For Women

Meal plan week 12

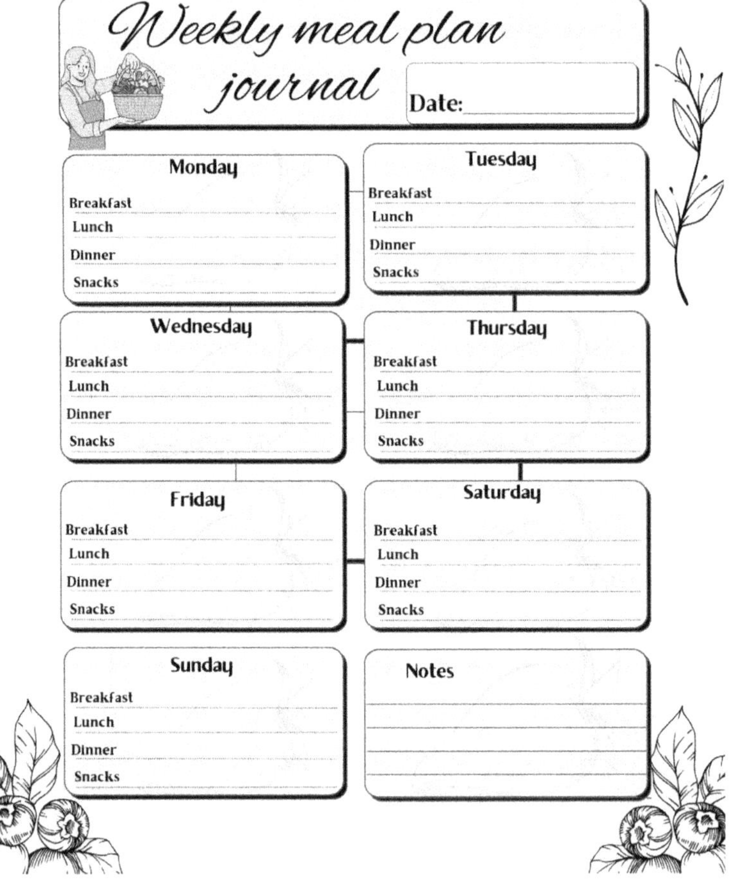

* 9 7 9 8 8 7 1 9 3 5 8 5 9 *